• SEO-HEE PARK •

Pilates at home

Achieve Flexibility,
Strength, and Balance
with Easy 15-, 30-, and
50-Minute Routines

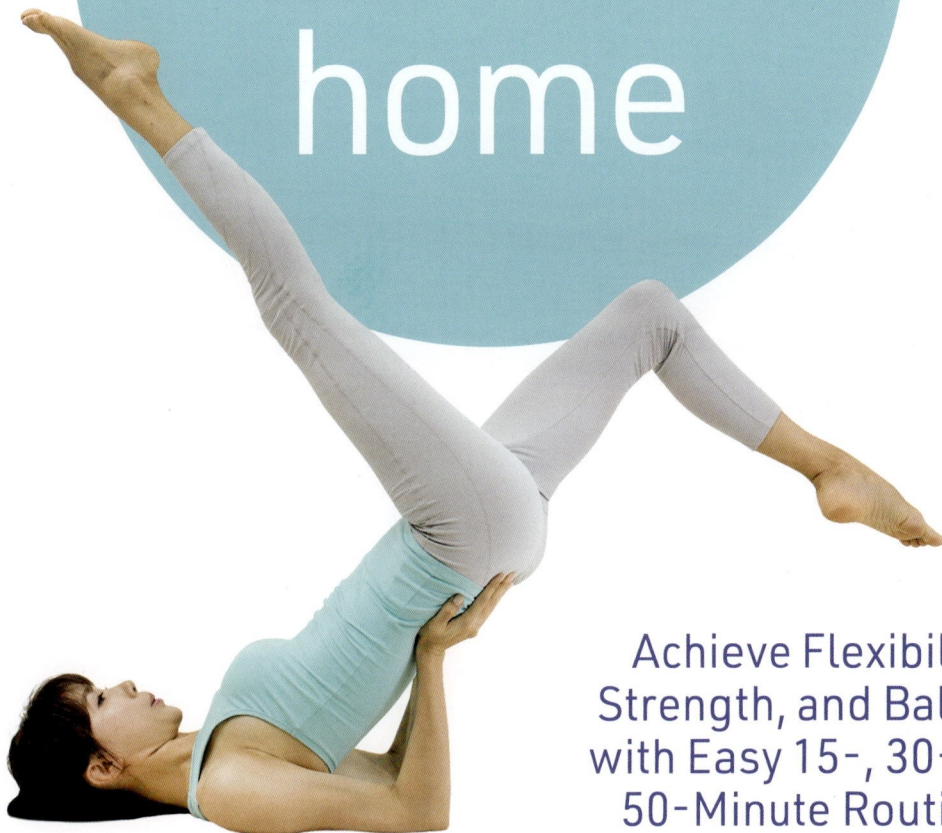

VELO
press®

Contents

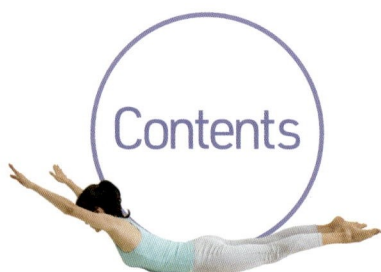

Part 1

Pilates Daily Program

Part 2

Pilates at Home

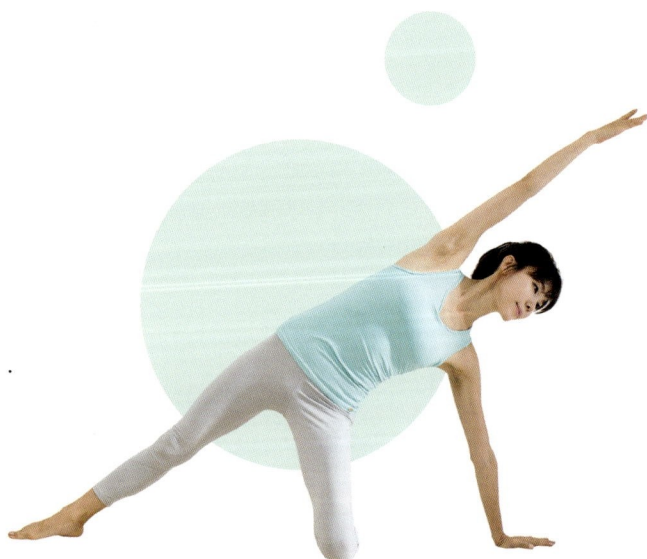

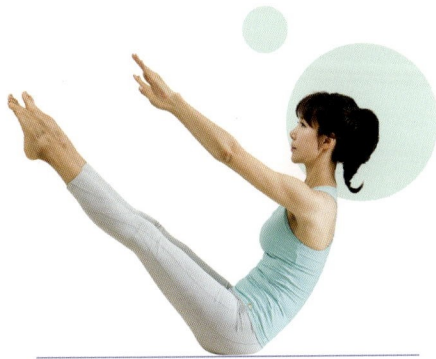

Part 3
Pilates with Props

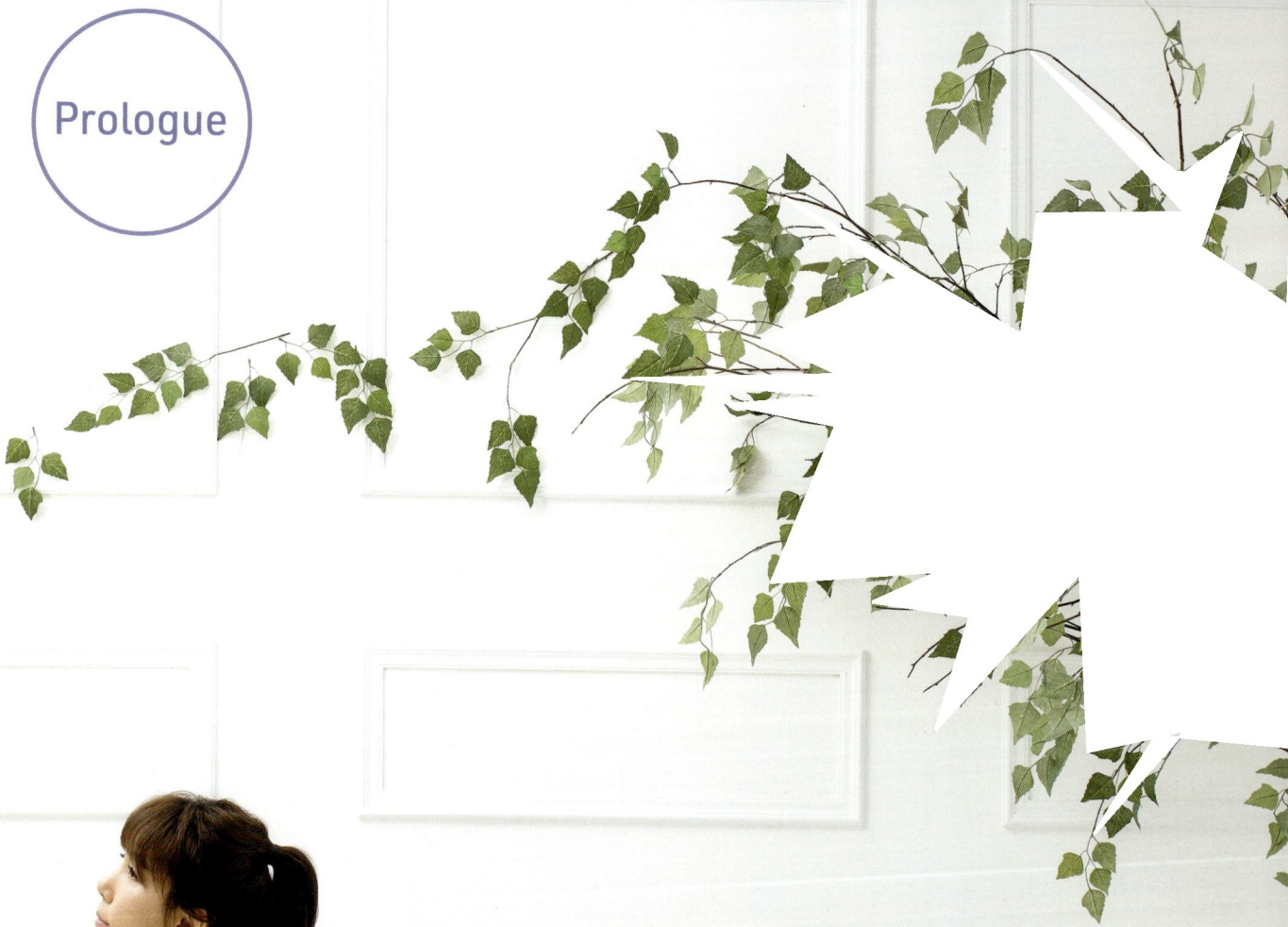

Prologue

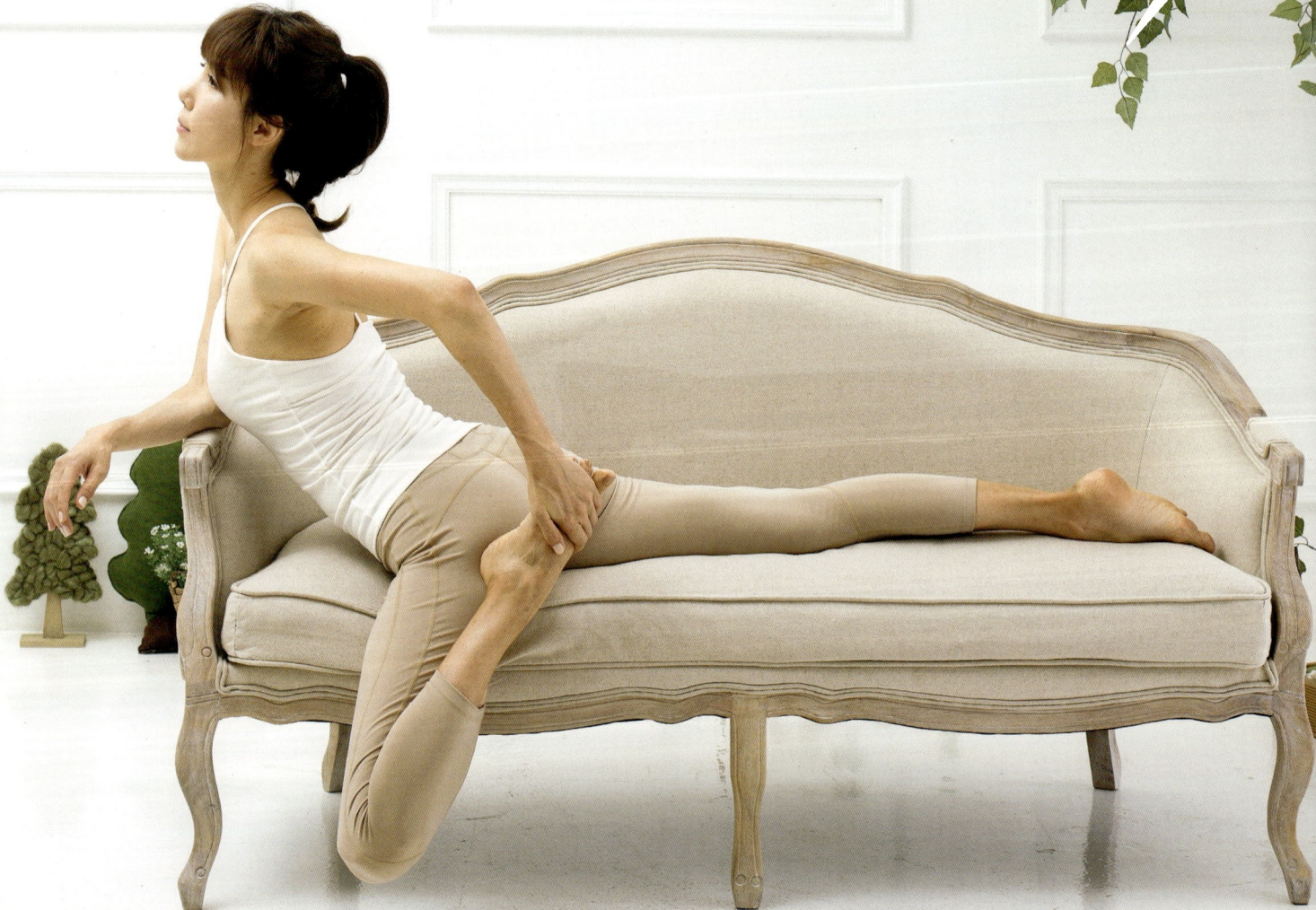

Pilates at Home

Pilates, which is usually associated with dancers and athletes, often begs the question, "Will I get in shape if I try it?" And the answer is a resounding yes. Pilates is not just for the already fit—it's a great full-body workout for anyone who wants to improve balance, muscle strength, and flexibility. Plus, if you practice Pilates regularly, you'll lose excess flab by building your muscles and improve your body's balance by strengthening your joints and spine.

Pilates can also help relieve stress and improve cardiovascular fitness. While it shares many similarities with yoga—both enhance muscular strength, endurance, and flexibility—Pilates is a more active exercise, enabling greater weight loss with more vigorous workout sessions.

Invented by German therapist Joseph H. Pilates during World War II as a therapeutic rehabilitation method for recovering soldiers, Pilates is scientifically based on the human anatomy and designed to strengthen the body's core muscles. The essence of Pilates is to tense and relax the body's muscles steadily and repeatedly. This strengthens sensitive muscles and joints while improving overall flexibility rather than straining the body.

Pilates often utilizes various exercise tools such as foam rollers, rings, gym balls, and resistance bands for optimum results. Yet, it's a common misconception that Pilates is an expensive exercise and is only available in professional studios. In reality, Pilates is one of the most cost-effective exercises available. It is a full-body workout that can be practiced anywhere at any time, with as much or as little gear as you like. *Pilates at Home*, an all-levels comprehensive guide for effortless Pilates, contains essential movements based on Joseph Pilates's principles, and the various workout options can be catered to one's fitness level, lifestyle, and schedule.

So, grab a mat and start your personalized fitness journey with *Pilates at Home*!

Seo-Hee Park

PILATES
How to Use This Book

Depending on how much time you have, you can choose between 15-, 30-, or 50-minute workout programs.

I have organized the workouts based on posture to provide practical training for each part of your body.

Detailed instructions for each of 15-, 30-, or 50-minute workouts are provided.

Method and number of repetitions are provided for each movement.

Precautions and additional information about the exercises are provided.

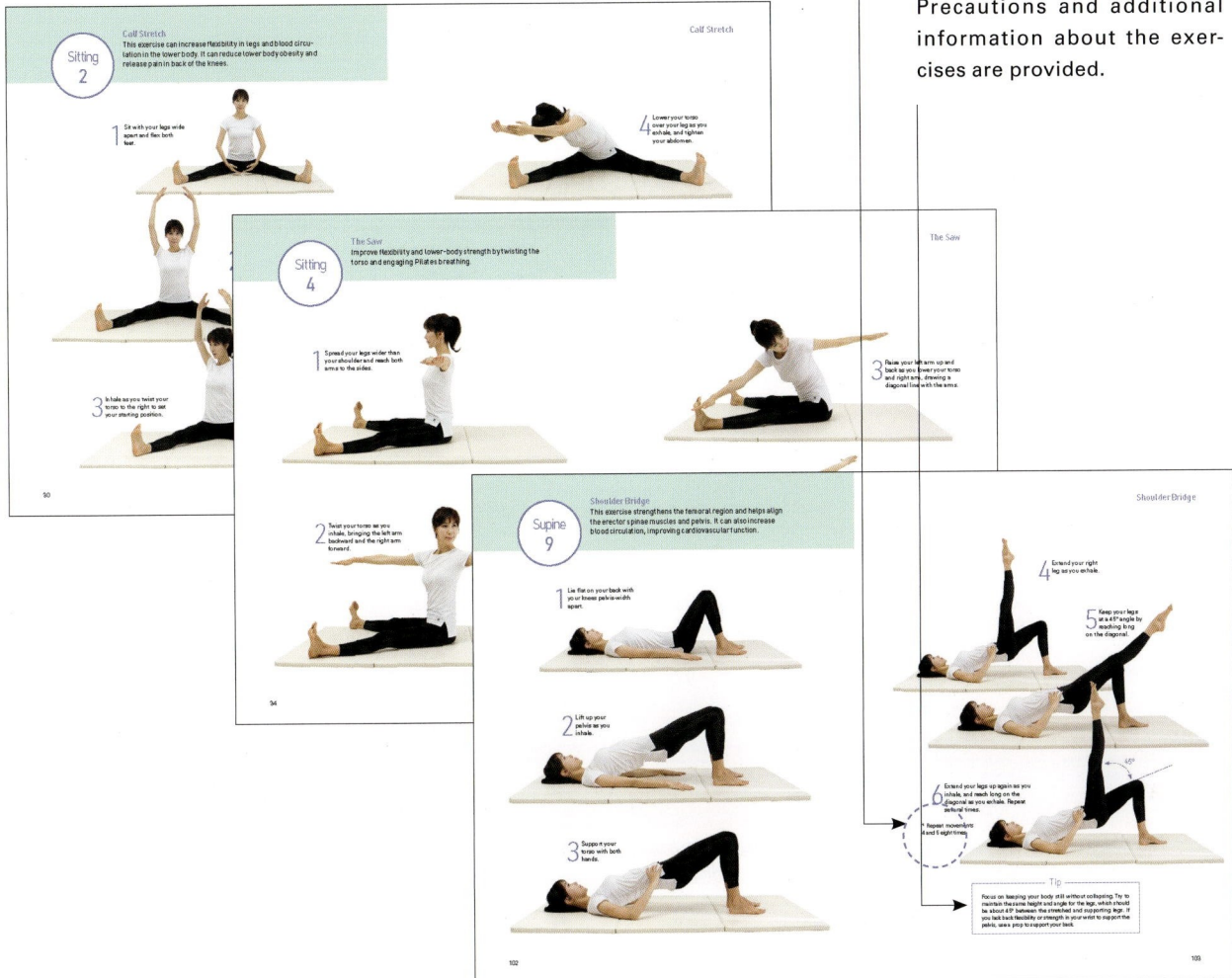

How to use this book for the best results:

1 Go through the book from beginning to end.

2 Practice the 15-minute program for a week.

3 Practice the 30-minute program for a month.

4 Practice the 50-minute program according to your own DIY workout plan.

5 Cut out the images from the book according to your DIY workout and place the images where you can easily see them.

NEUTRAL POSTURE
The Basic Pilates Posture

Maintaining a neutral posture is one of the most essential principles in Pilates. Try to hold the correct posture focusing on the powerhouse, which is the core center of energy and control. Practice your standing, supine, and sitting postures to master the foundation of every movement.

Standing Neutral

Stretch your spine and stand upright with your ears, shoulders, pelvis, and knees in a straight line. Check your posture regularly.

How to stand upright

Stand with your feet a comfortable distance apart and open your chest wide. Stretch your shoulders and bring your chin toward your body. Tighten your thighs and hips and tuck your stomach in.

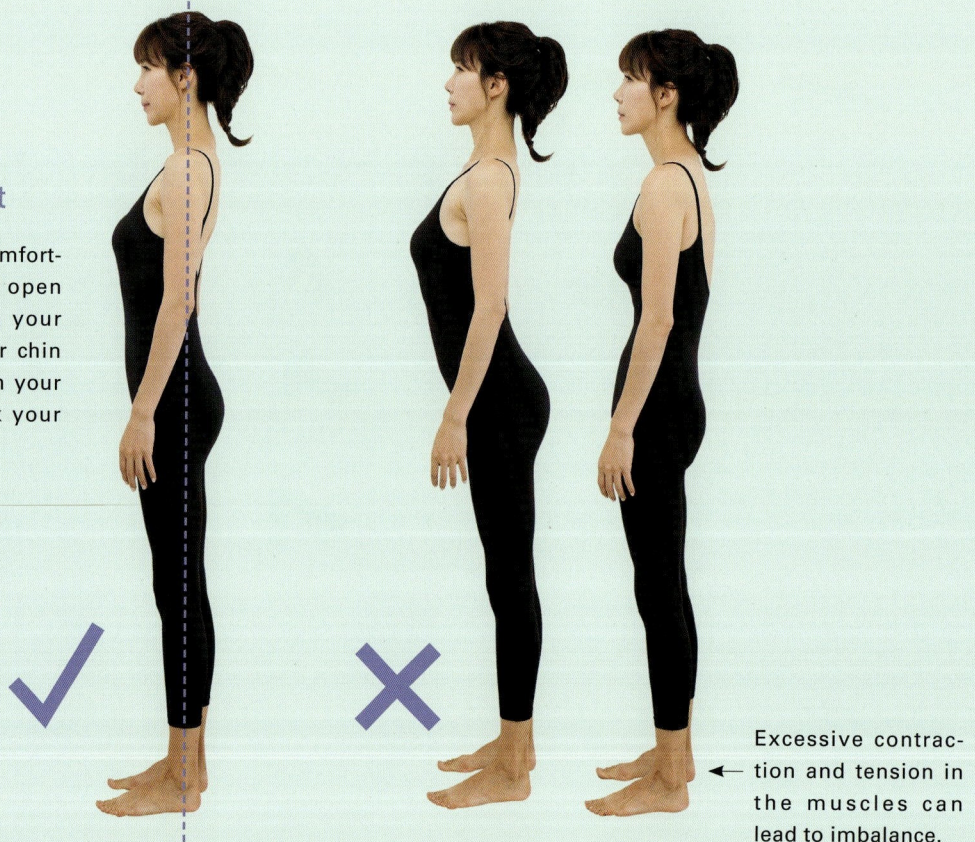

Excessive contraction and tension in the muscles can lead to imbalance.

Basics of Pilates Core, Powerhouse, and Breathing

The powerhouse and core are the fundamental concepts of Pilates.

The core is the center of the body, which enables all movement. The abdominal, back, and hip muscles are the core muscles. The core connects the lumbar, pelvis, and hips while also connecting the center of the body. Strong core muscles can better support the spine, and a stronger spine can make the entire body more robust, strengthening the muscles and improving overall power.

The core is also referred to as the "powerhouse" because it's the source of energy. In order to correct the spine, you need to exercise the powerhouse.

Another important concept of Pilates is breathing. Each Pilates movement has its own breathing cycles, and the best results are obtained when following the cycles. Try to concentrate throughout each movement and steadily connect each step, following the flow.

Supine Neutral

Lie flat on your back from head to toe. Maintain the natural arch of your neck and back. Keep your feet parallel, with your toes pointing slightly outward. .

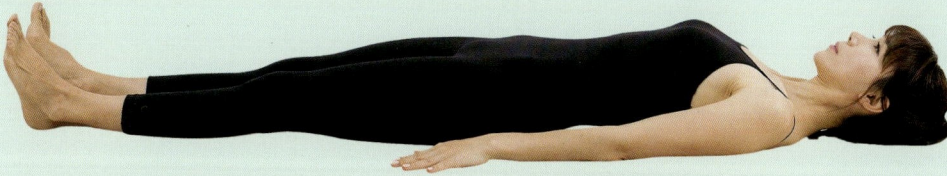

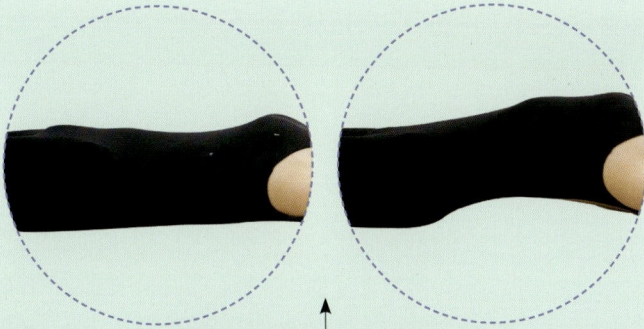

Correct supine pose

Lie flat on your back with your toes comfortably spread. Ease your shoulders and tuck your chin. Breathe out to make your chest flat and try to maintain the natural curve of your body to keep your posture neutral between the floor and your back.

Excessive muscle contraction and tension can disrupt the natural curve of the back.

Sitting Neutral

Make sure your legs and back are perpendicular to your hips. Keep your legs fully stretched and flat on the floor.

Correct sitting pose

Sit with your legs and spine stretched straight. Make a 90° angle between your legs and back. Tuck your chin and make a straight line through your ears, shoulders, and pelvis. Flex your feet.

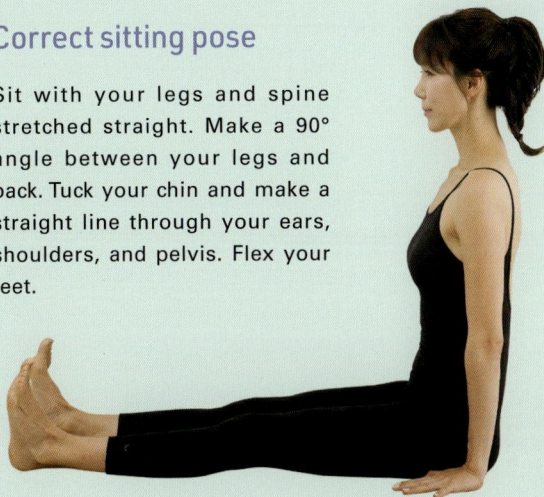

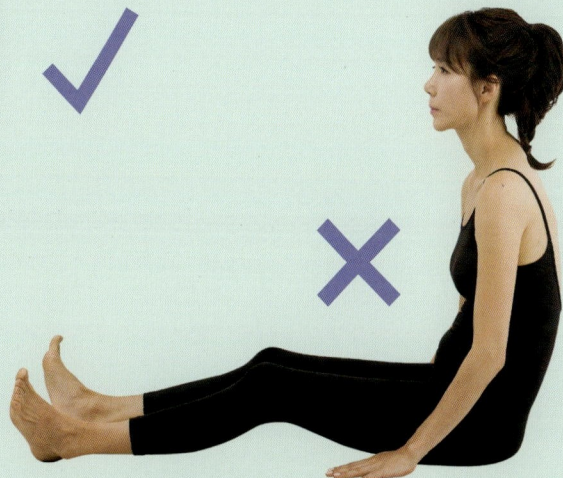

Be conscious of your core.

Daily Pilates Program

It's important to practice Pilates routinely because the basic concept is to tense and relax the muscles repeatedly. Depending on your condition and fitness level, select between 15-, 30-, and 50-minute programs. If you exercise every day on a regular basis, you will lose excess flab and become more fit.

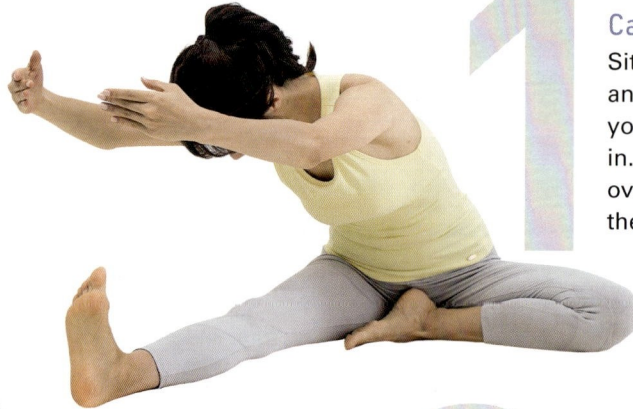

1 Calf Stretch

Sit with one leg extended and flex your foot toward you. Bend the other leg in. Stretch your arms overhead and bend over the extended leg. (See p. 31)

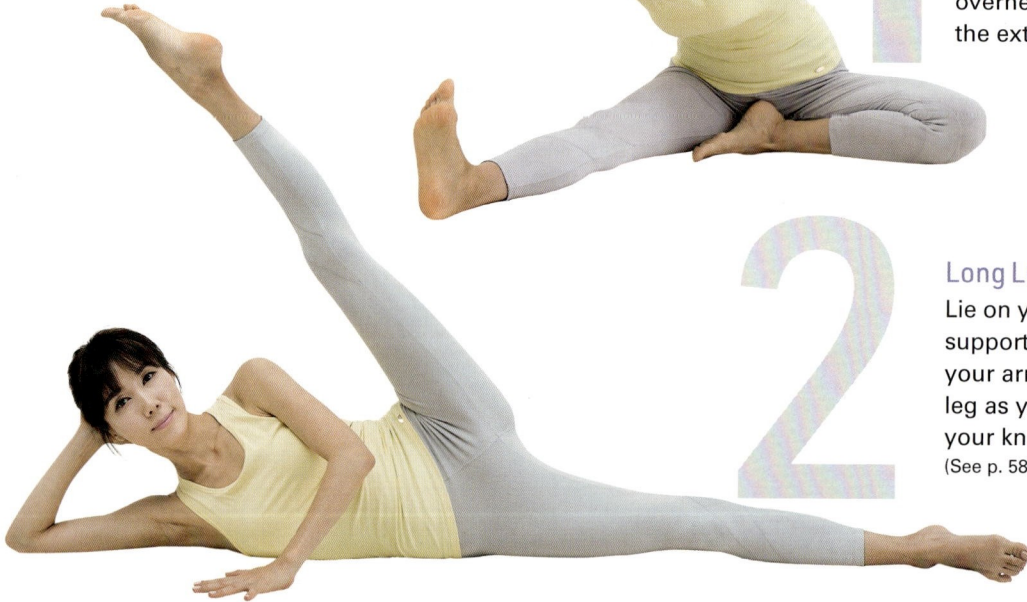

2 Long Leg Lift

Lie on your right side and support your head with your arm. Raise your left leg as you inhale. Bend your knee as you exhale. (See p. 58)

3 The Sphinx

Lie on your belly with your legs pelvis-width apart and place your forearms on the floor. Lift your torso to the sphinx position and then round down and relax your spine. (See p. 62)

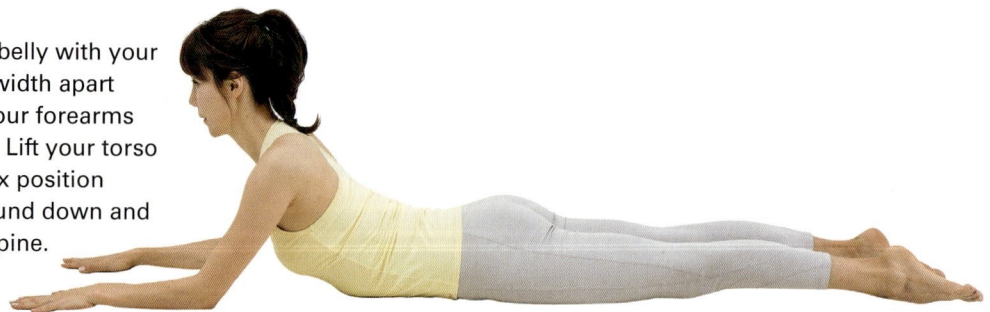

4 Swimming

Lie on your belly with both arms reaching forward. Lift up your right arm and left leg, then left arm and right leg, repeatedly, as if you were swimming. (See p. 66)

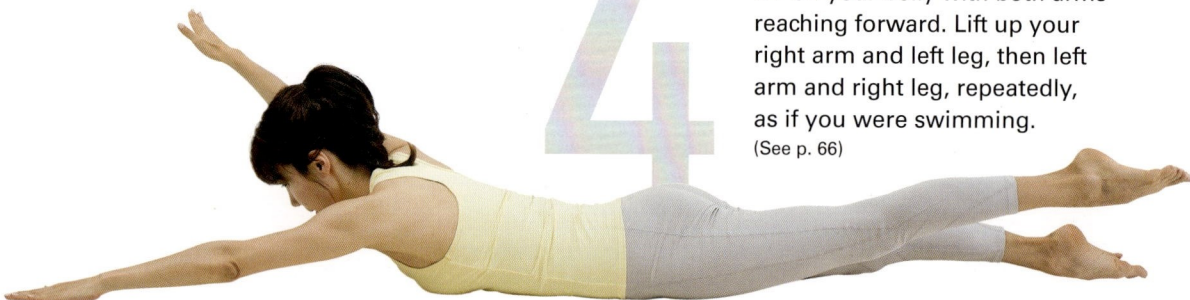

5 Leg Kick-Back

Start on all fours, then kick one leg back. Bend the knee and bring the leg in toward the chest, then kick back again. (See p. 78)

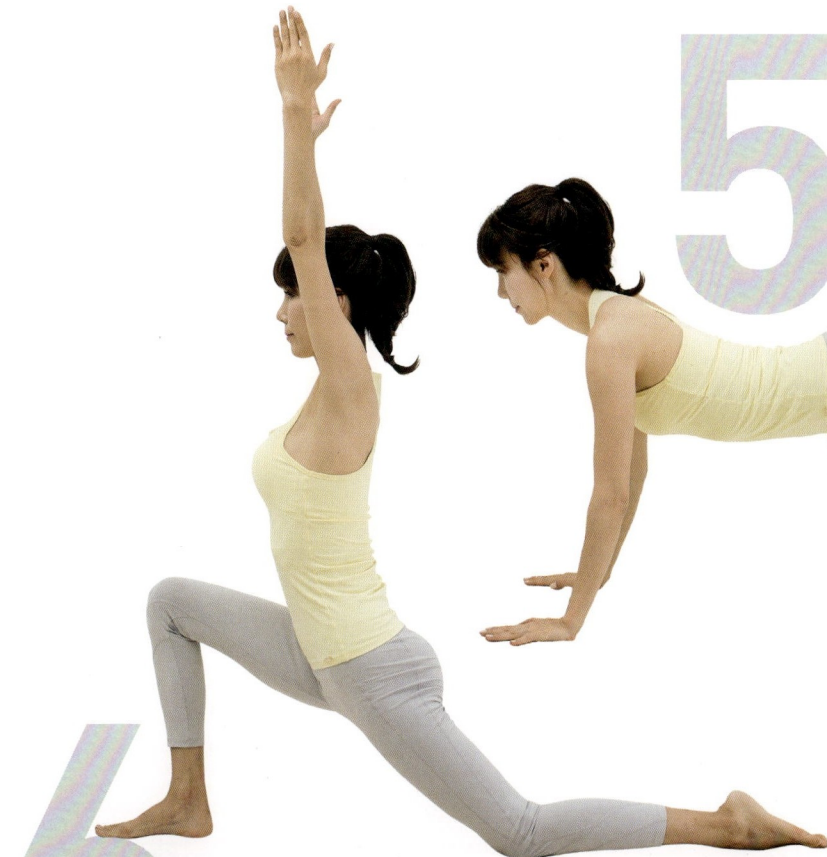

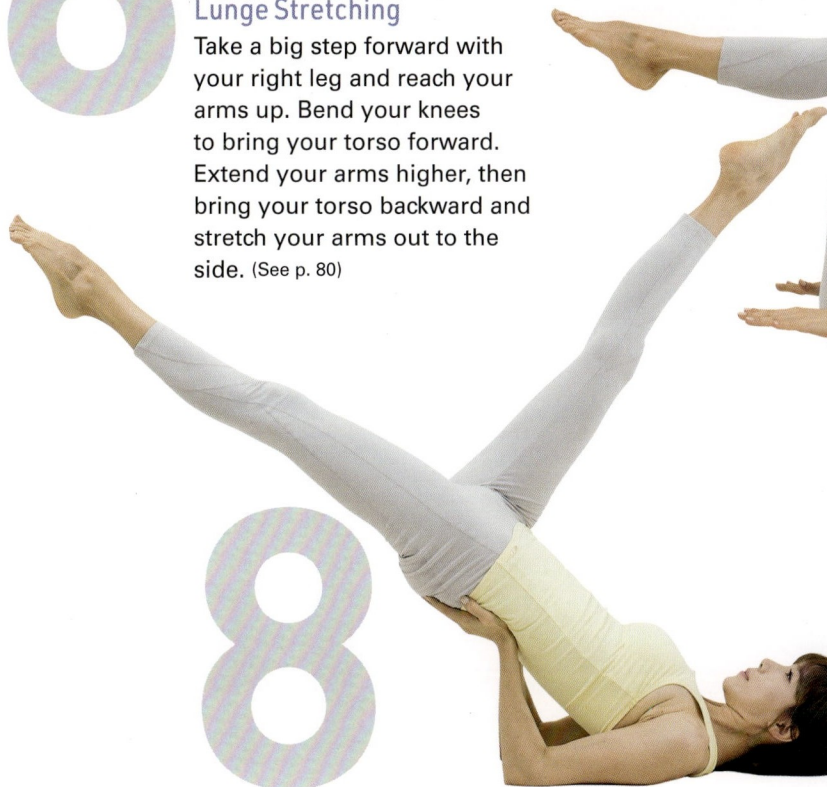

6 Lunge Stretching

Take a big step forward with your right leg and reach your arms up. Bend your knees to bring your torso forward. Extend your arms higher, then bring your torso backward and stretch your arms out to the side. (See p. 80)

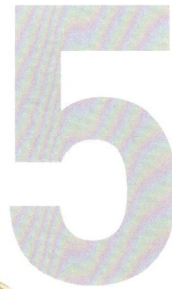

7 The Hundred

Lie on your back with your knees bent at 90° and lift up your torso. Extend your arms by your sides and breath out in short spurts while pumping your arms up and down. (See p. 90)

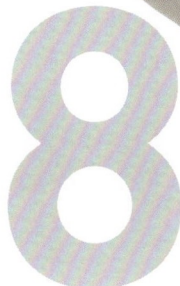

8 The Scissors

Supporting your torso with both arms, extend and raise your legs. Stretch your legs back and forth like scissors. (See p. 100)

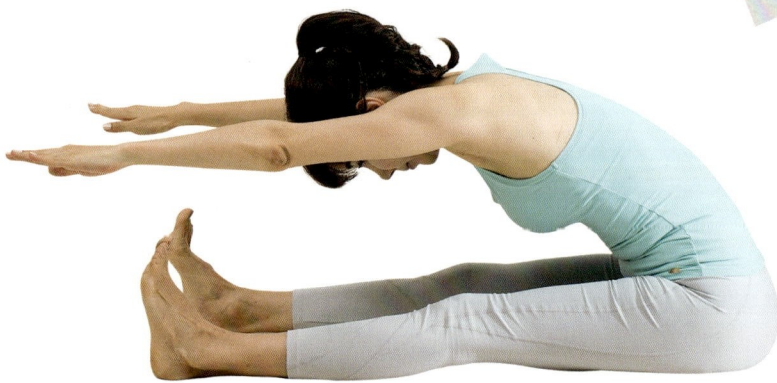

1

Spine Stretch Forward

Sit with your spine straight and your legs shoulder-width apart and flex your feet. Raise your arms, then bend your arms and torso forward as deeply as you can. (See p. 28)

The Teaser

Start in a seated position and lift your legs off the ground, extending them straight out in front of you. Stretch your arms forward, keeping them parallel to your legs. (See p. 36)

2

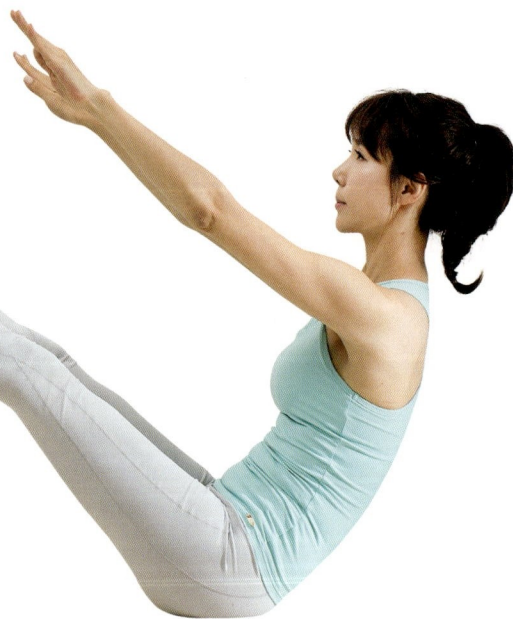

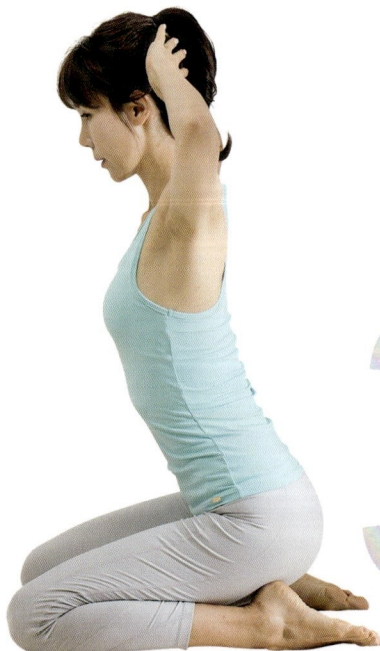

3

Kneeling Squat

Start in a kneeling position, then rise up onto your knees and twist your torso to the right. Return to the starting position, then rise up and twist to the opposite side. (See p. 42)

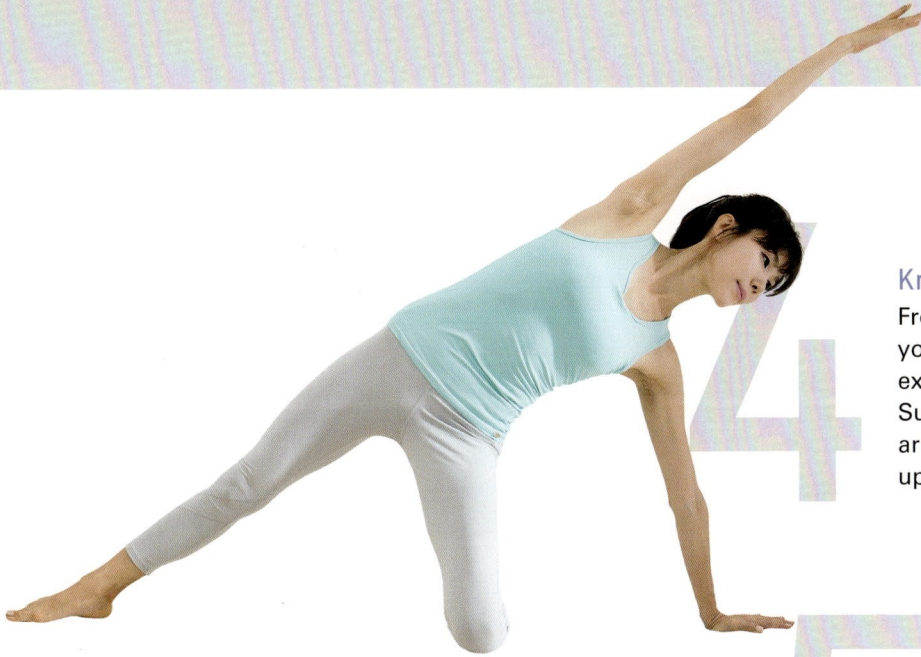

Kneeling Side Bend

From a kneeling position, lean your body to the left side and extend your right arm and right leg. Support your body with your left arm and left leg and lift your body up and down. (See p. 46)

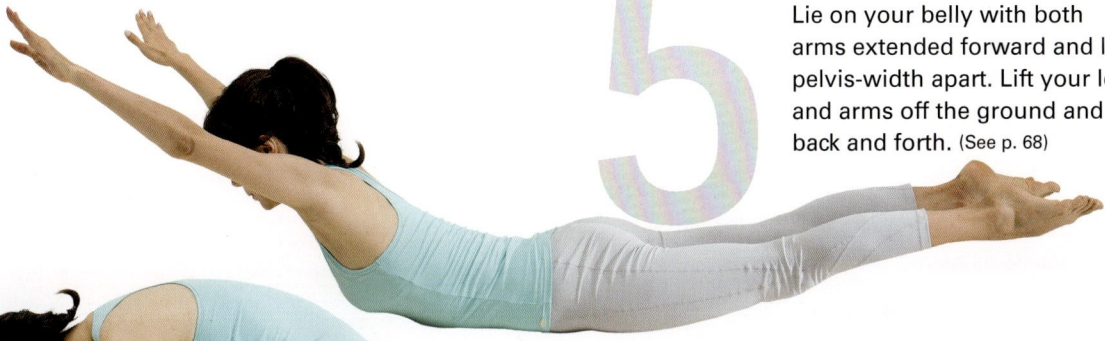

The Swan

Lie on your belly with both arms extended forward and legs pelvis-width apart. Lift your legs and arms off the ground and rock back and forth. (See p. 68)

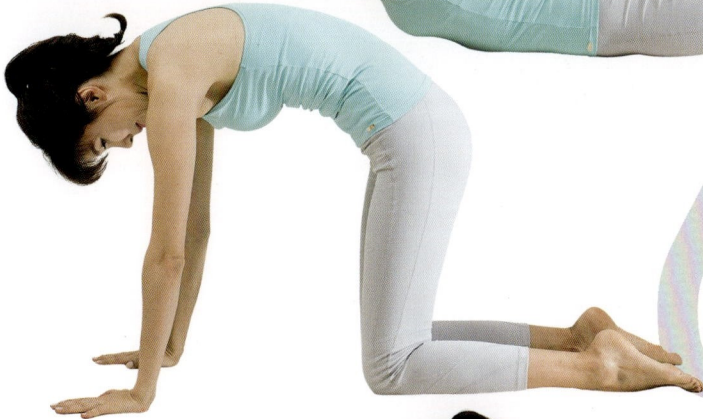

Cat Stretch

Start in the all-fours position. Round your spine and head down, then round your torso and head up. (See p. 74)

Leg Pull–Front

From the push-up position, keeping a diagonal line from head to toe, alternate lifting each leg. (See p. 82)

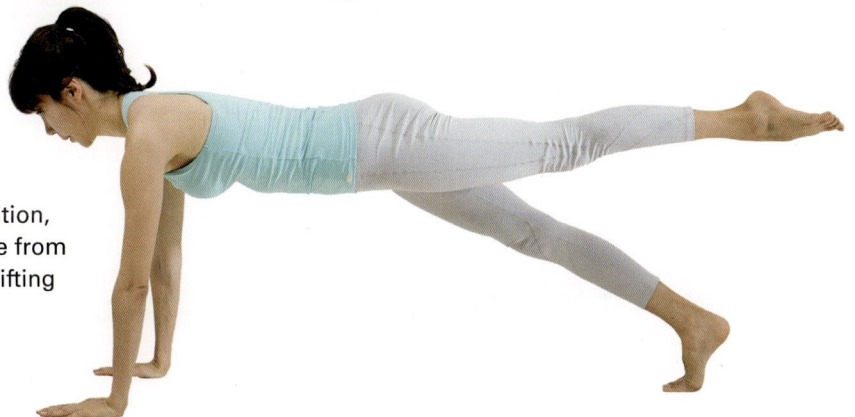

8

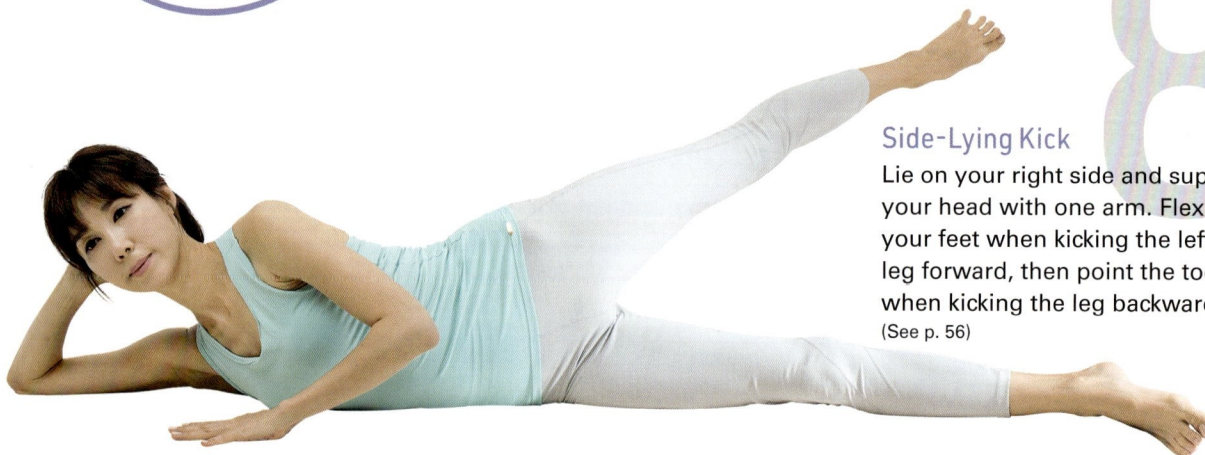

Side-Lying Kick

Lie on your right side and support your head with one arm. Flex your feet when kicking the left leg forward, then point the toes when kicking the leg backward. (See p. 56)

9

One-Leg Stretch

Lie on your back and bring your right knee toward your chest. Curl up your torso and extend your left leg in a diagonal line. (See p. 88)

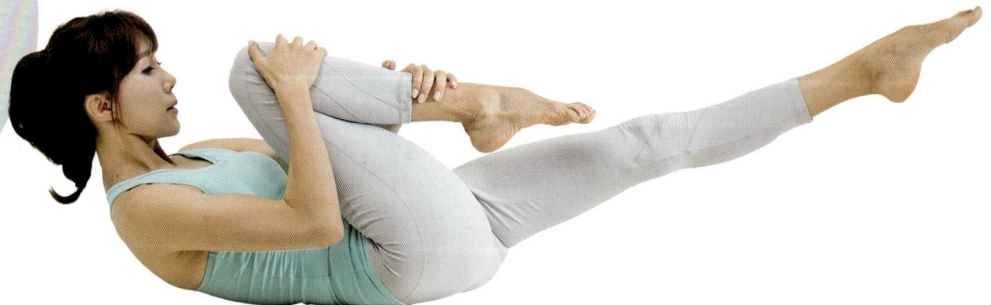

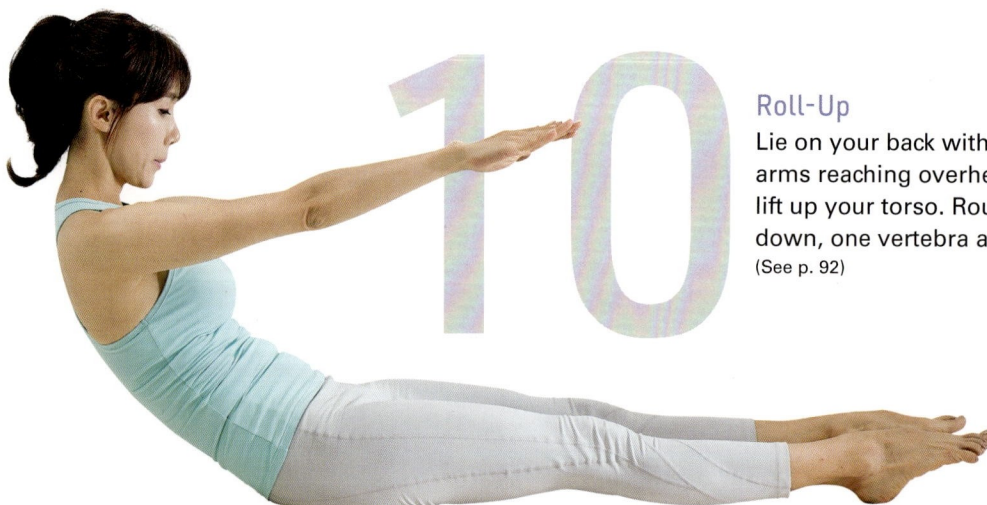

10

Roll-Up

Lie on your back with both arms reaching overhead and lift up your torso. Round back down, one vertebra at a time. (See p. 92)

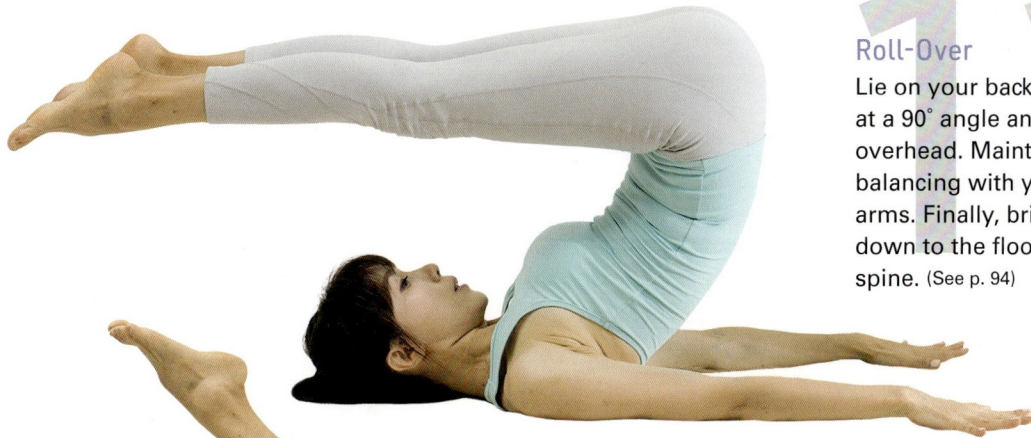

11 Roll-Over

Lie on your back with your knees bent at a 90° angle and bring both legs overhead. Maintain the posture by balancing with your shoulders and arms. Finally, bring your legs slowly down to the floor, rounding your spine. (See p. 94)

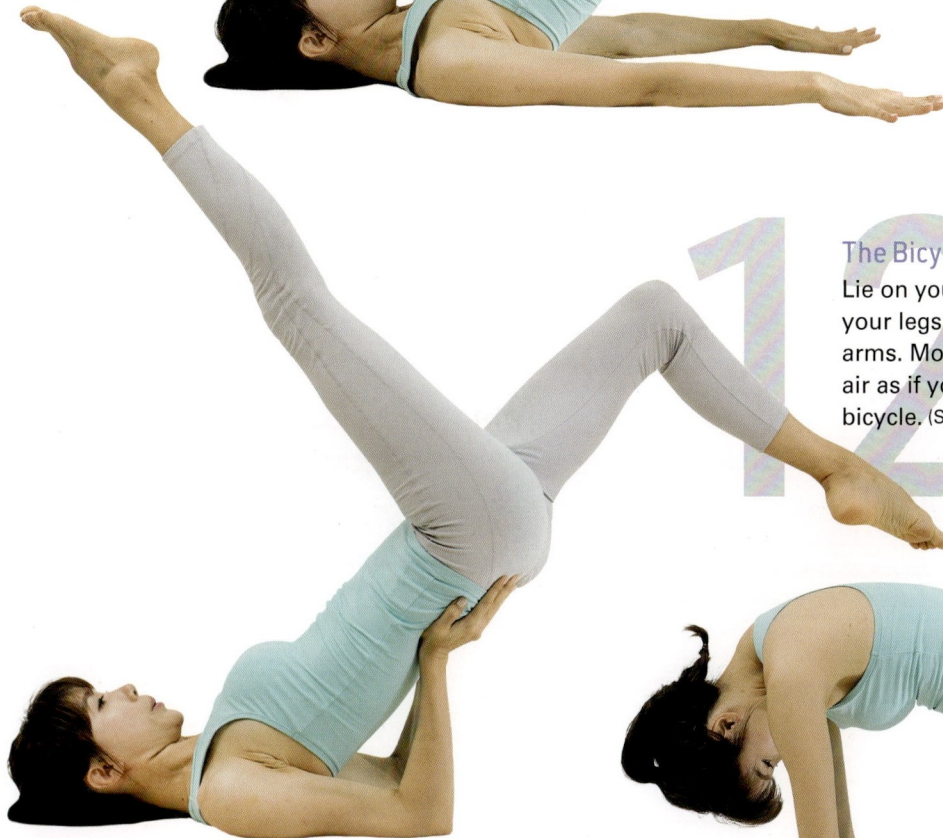

12 The Bicycle

Lie on your back and support your legs and body with your arms. Move your legs in the air as if you were pedaling a bicycle. (See p. 96)

13 Standing Roll-Down

Stand straight with your feet pelvis-width apart. Slowly bend your head down with your arms relaxed. Stop before your hands touch the ground. (See p. 108)

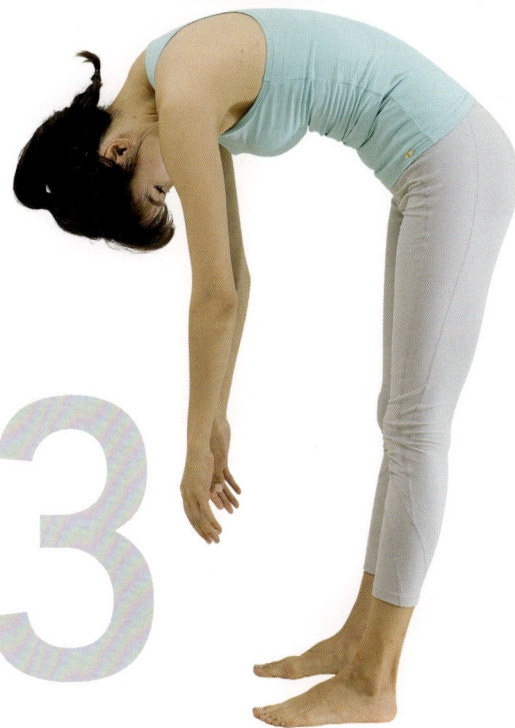

1

Spine Twist

Sit with your legs wide apart and feet flexed. Reach your arms to the sides with your spine straight. Twist your torso, then return to the starting position and twist to the other side. (See p. 32)

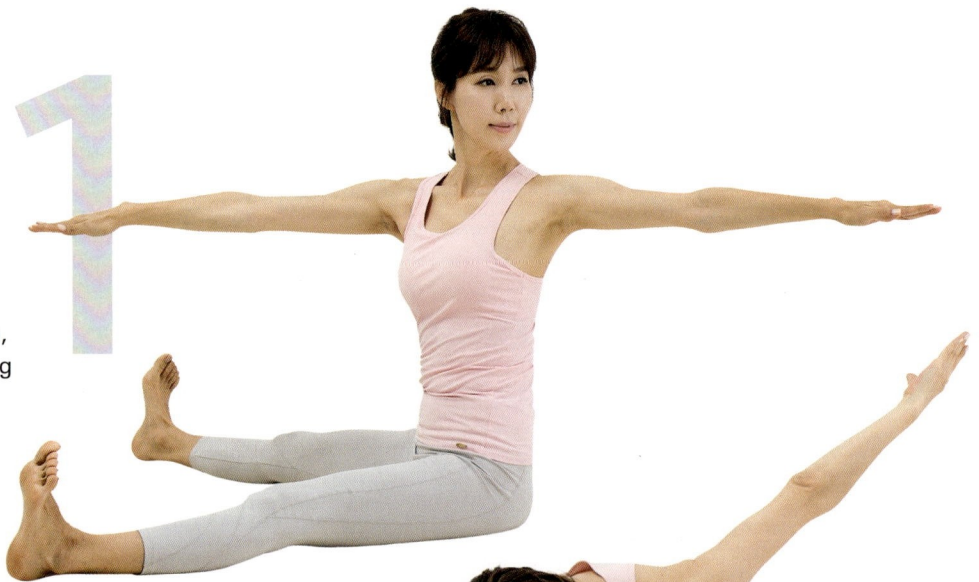

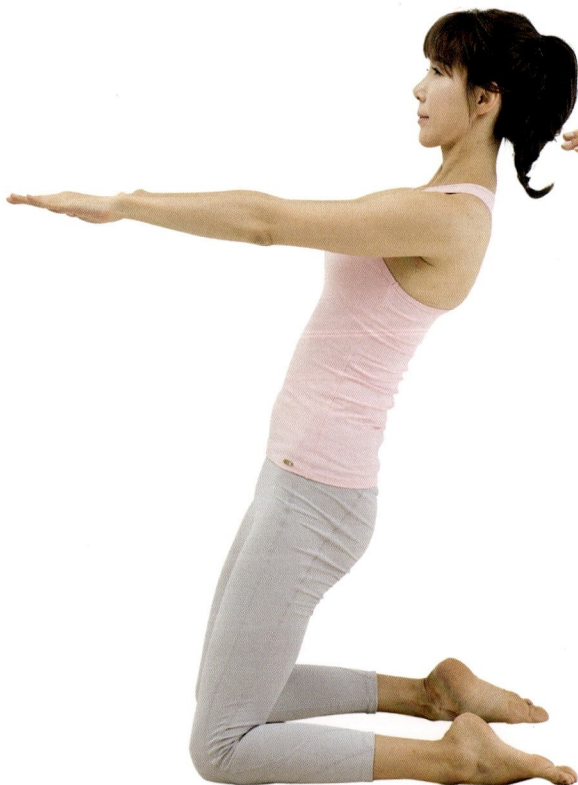

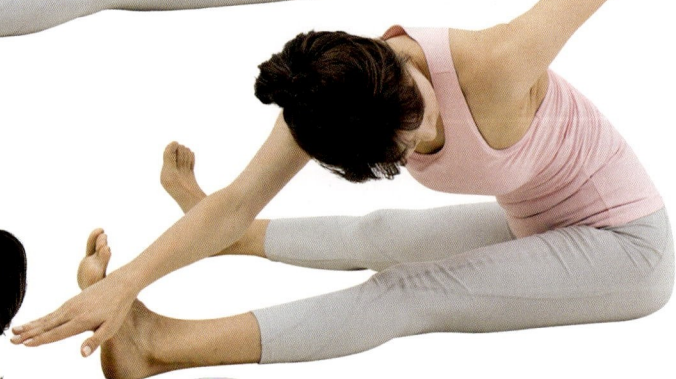

2

The Saw

Sit with your legs wider than your shoulders. Reach your arms to the sides. Bend forward while twisting your torso, raising the left arm up and back and lowering the right arm forward. (See p. 34)

3

Thigh Stretching

Stand on your knees with your legs shoulder-width apart and reach your arms forward. Slowly lower your torso backward. (See p. 40)

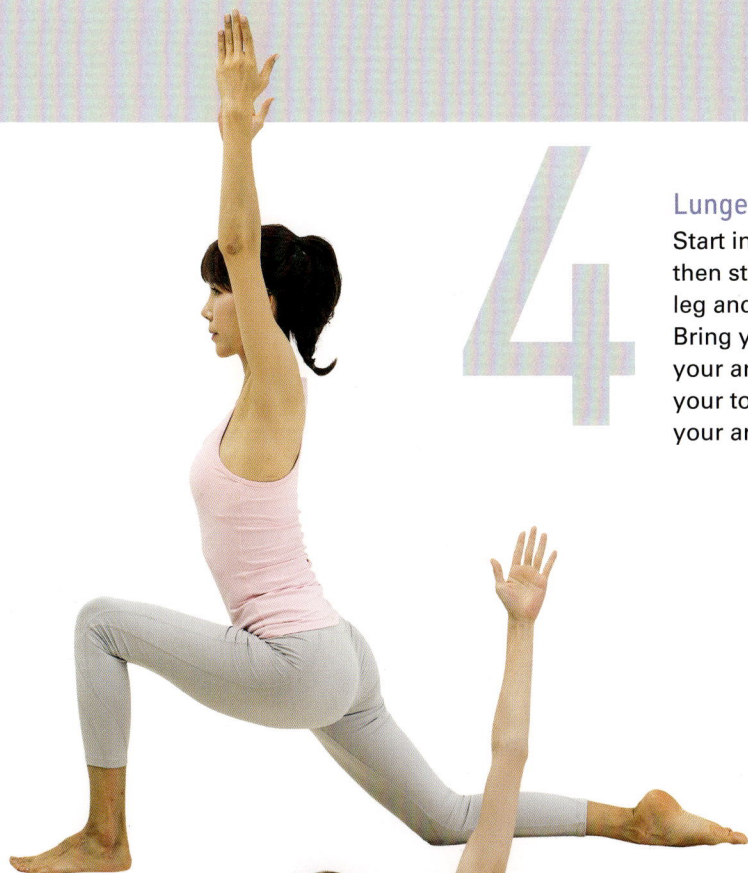

Lunge Stretching

Start in the all-fours position, then step forward with your left leg and reach your arms up. Bring your torso forward. Extend your arms higher, then bring your torso backward and stretch your arms to the side. (See p. 80)

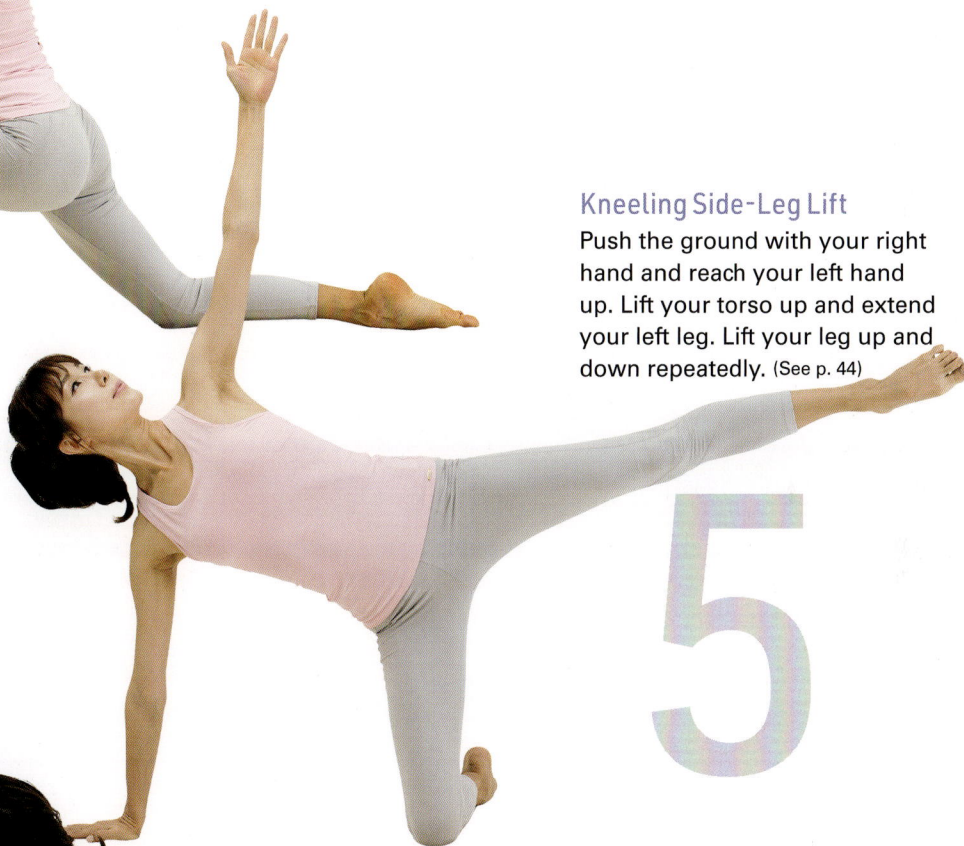

Kneeling Side-Leg Lift

Push the ground with your right hand and reach your left hand up. Lift your torso up and extend your left leg. Lift your leg up and down repeatedly. (See p. 44)

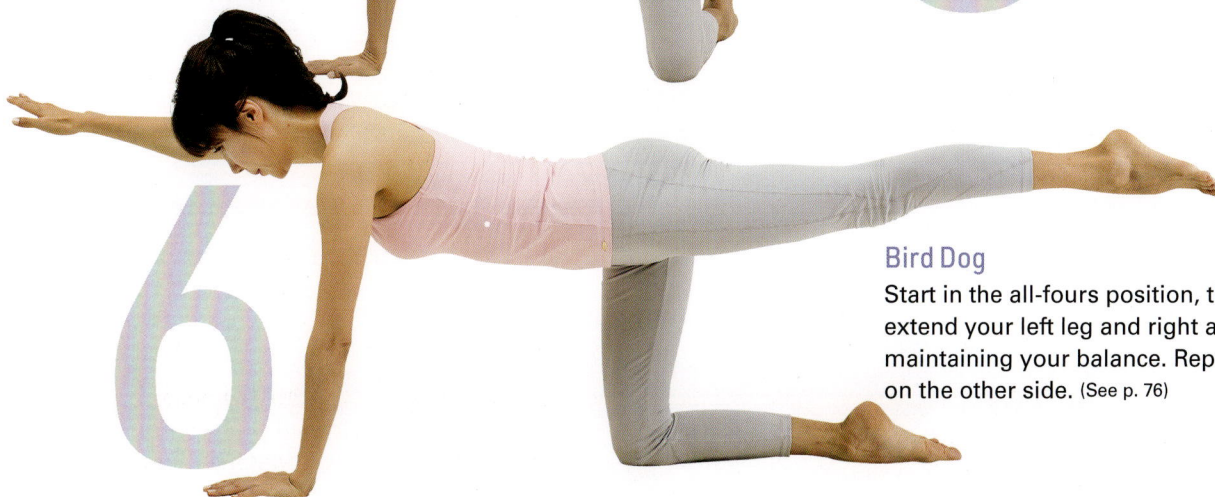

Bird Dog

Start in the all-fours position, then extend your left leg and right arm, maintaining your balance. Repeat on the other side. (See p. 76)

7

Leg Raise

Lie on your belly with your hands placed under your forehead. Tighten your abdomen and lift your legs up and down without touching the floor. (See p. 64)

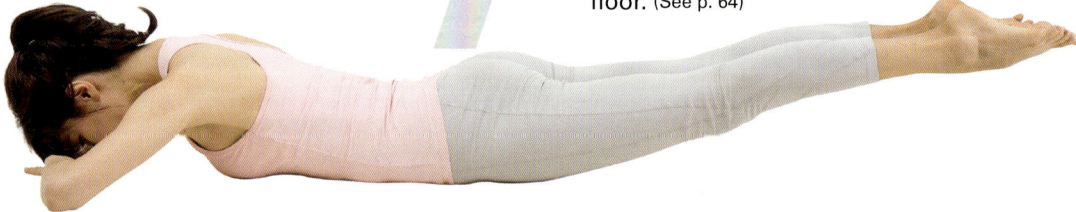

8

The Sphinx

Lie on your belly with your legs pelvis-width apart. Place your forearms on the floor in front of your chest. Lift your torso, then round and relax your spine. (See p. 62)

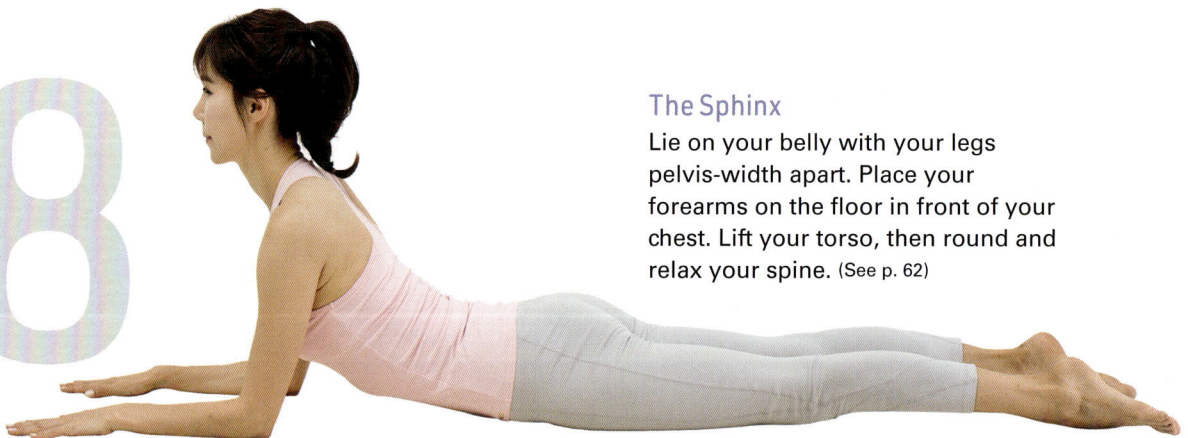

9

Double Kick

Lie on your belly with your hands placed under your forehead. Bend your knees and point and flex your feet. Then extend both legs and spread them wide. (See p. 70)

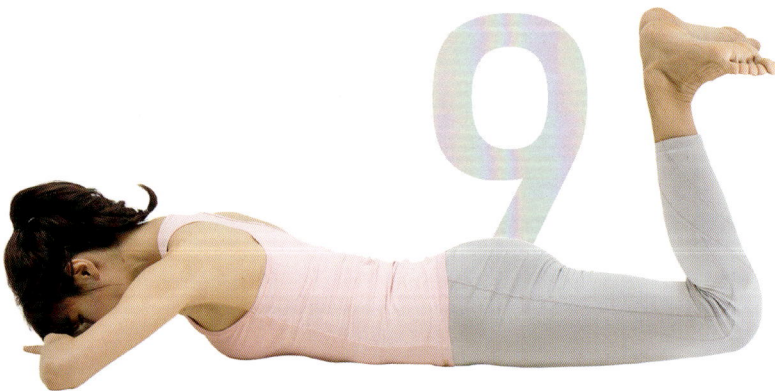

10

The Clam

Lie on your side and bend one arm to support your head. Bend your knees and tighten your glutes while lifting up your left knee, then return to the starting position and repeat. (See p. 50)

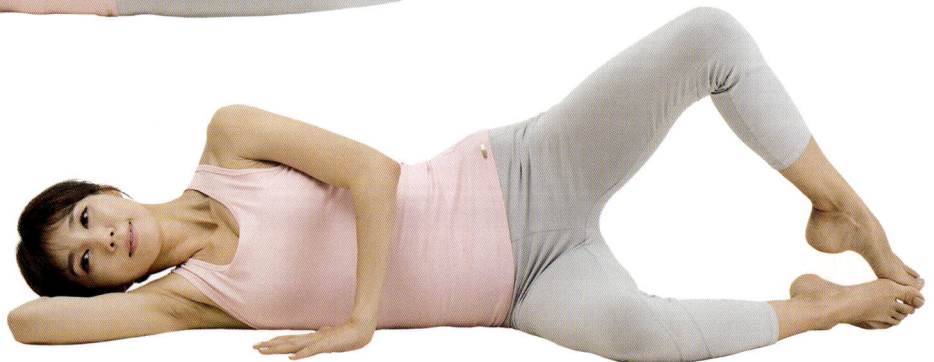

11

Side-Lying Leg Lift

Lie on your side with one arm bent to support your head and the other arm placed in front of your chest. Lift your leg up and down several times. (See p. 52)

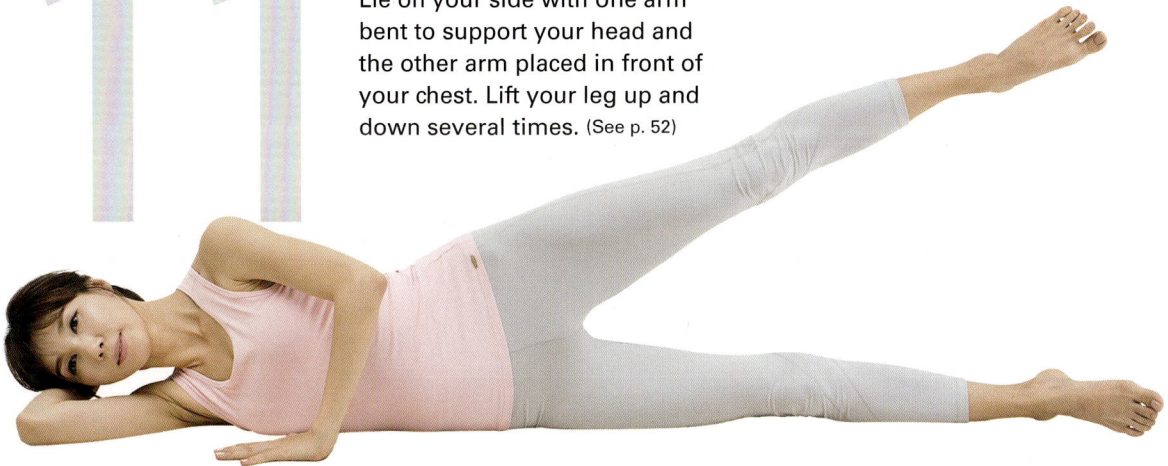

12

Inner Thigh Lift

Lie on your right side and support your head with your right hand. Hold your left ankle with your left hand and bring it to the floor. Lift the other leg up and down.
(See p. 54)

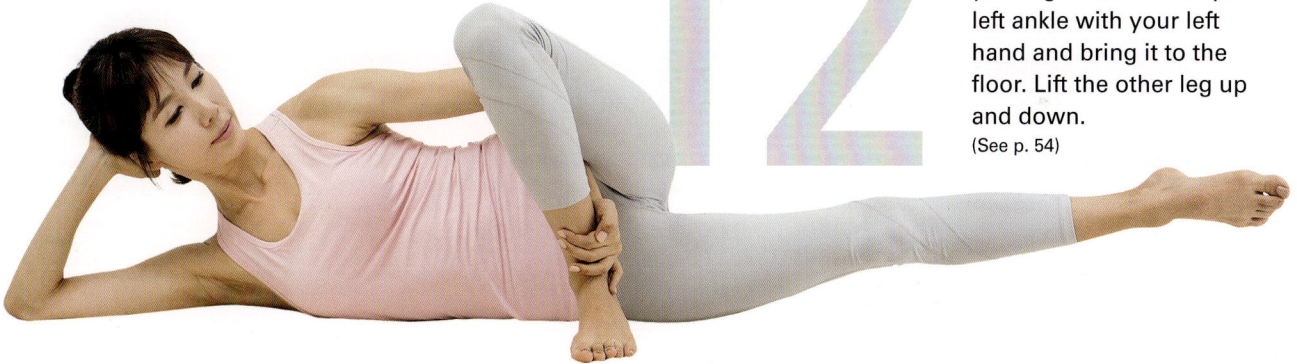

13

Leg Sliding

Lie on your back with your knees bent and rest your hands on your lower abdomen. Extend your leg.
(See p. 86)

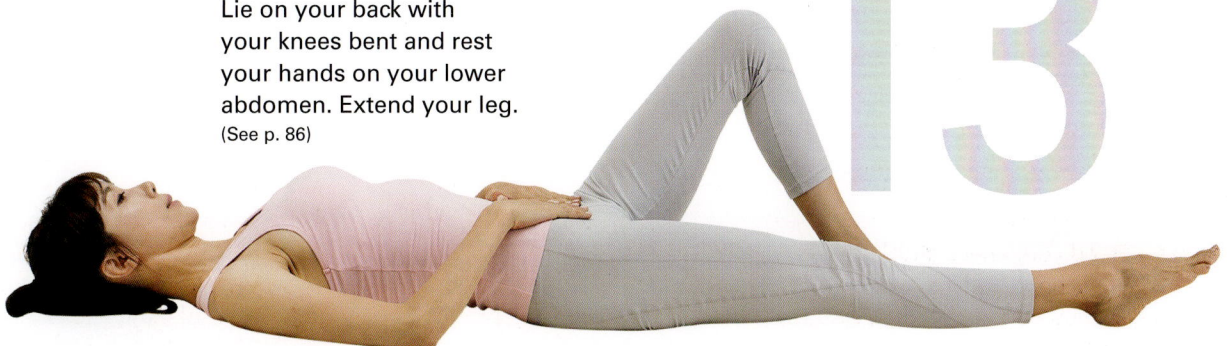

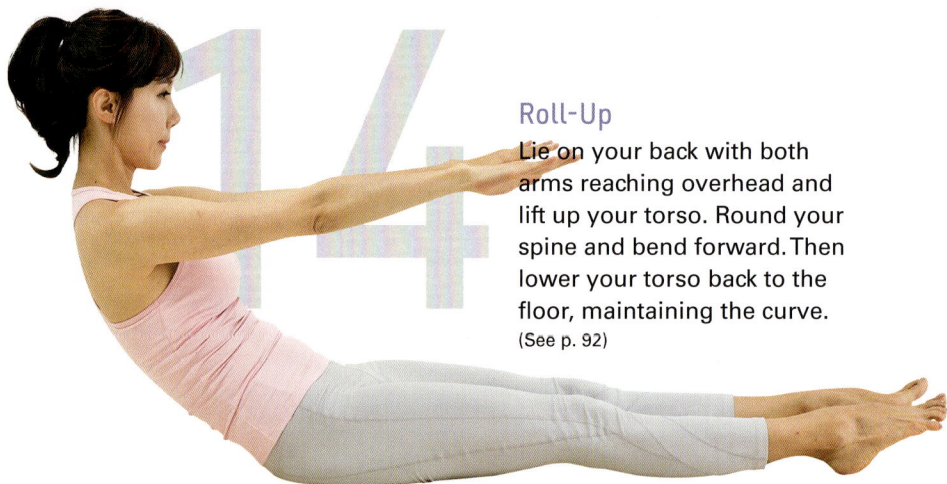

14 Roll-Up

Lie on your back with both arms reaching overhead and lift up your torso. Round your spine and bend forward. Then lower your torso back to the floor, maintaining the curve. (See p. 92)

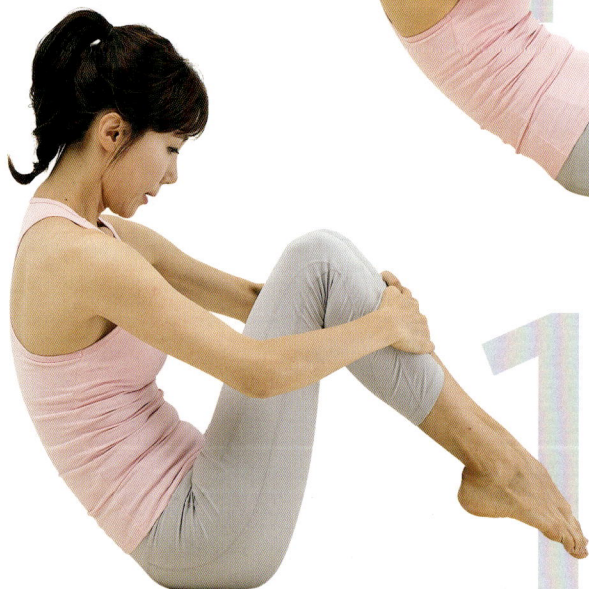

15 Rolling Back

Sit with your knees bent and hold your shins with your hands. Round your back and roll back and forth. (See p. 98)

16 The Hundred

Lie on your back with your arms and legs extended. Lift up your torso and legs and extend your arms by your sides. Breathe out in short spurts while pumping your arms up and down. (See p. 90)

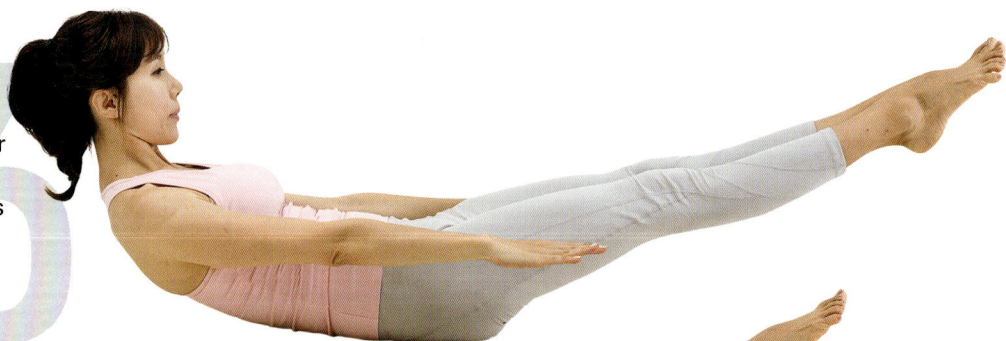

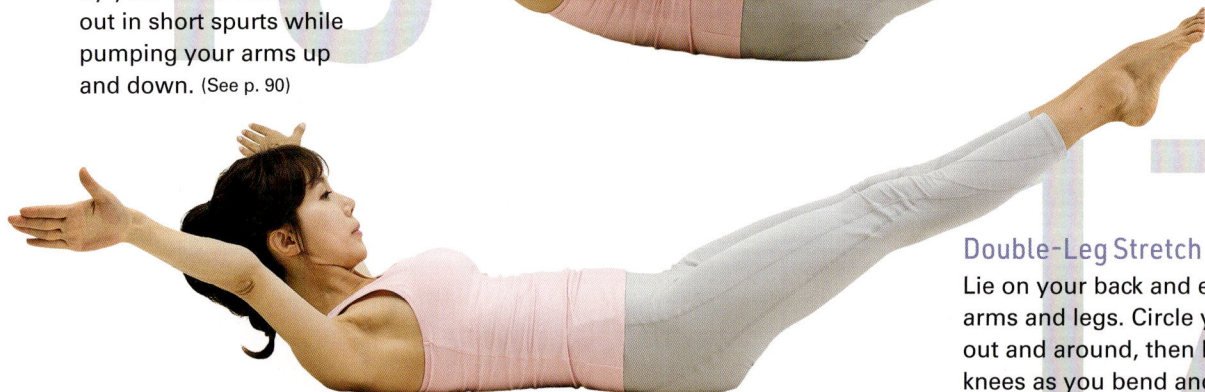

17 Double-Leg Stretch

Lie on your back and extend your arms and legs. Circle your arms out and around, then back to your knees as you bend and hold your knees. (See p. 104)

18

Shoulder Bridge

Lie on your back with both hands supporting your lower back and lift up your pelvis. Stretch one leg to a 45° angle. Raise the leg higher, then lower back to 45°. (See p. 102)

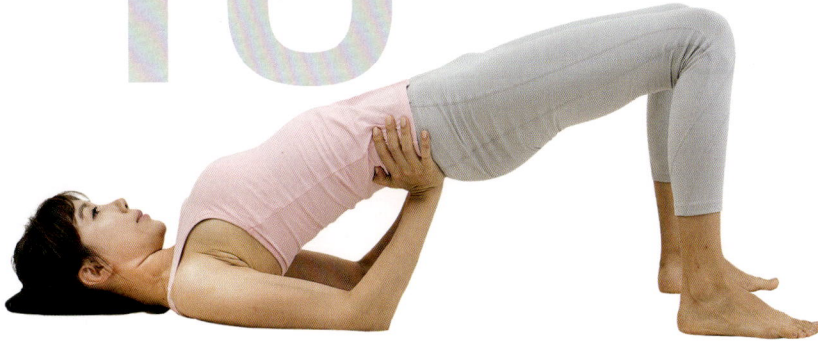

19

Standing Roll-Down

Stand straight with your feet pelvis-width apart. Slowly lower your head down with your hands relaxed. Stop before the hands touch the floor. (See p. 108)

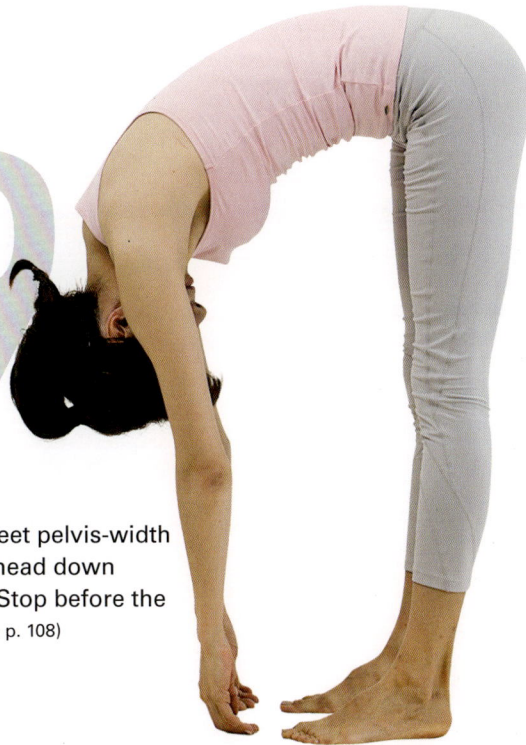

20

Pilates Breathing

Stand straight with your feet pelvis-width apart and bring your elbows together. Slowly raise your elbows above your head, opening your arms to draw a big circle as you lower them. (See p. 110)

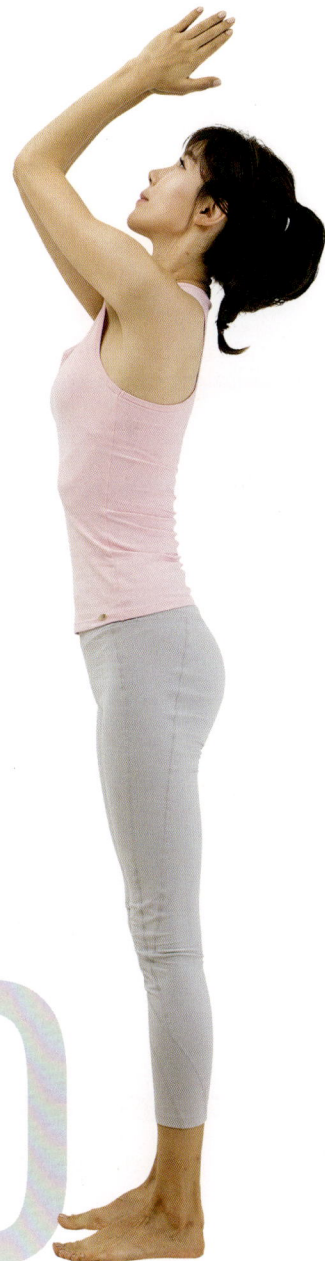

2

Pilates Home Training

Pilates is a full-body workout based on modern anatomy and exercise science. Once you familiarize yourself with the various movements for each position and body part, the daily program will maximize your workout results.

Sitting

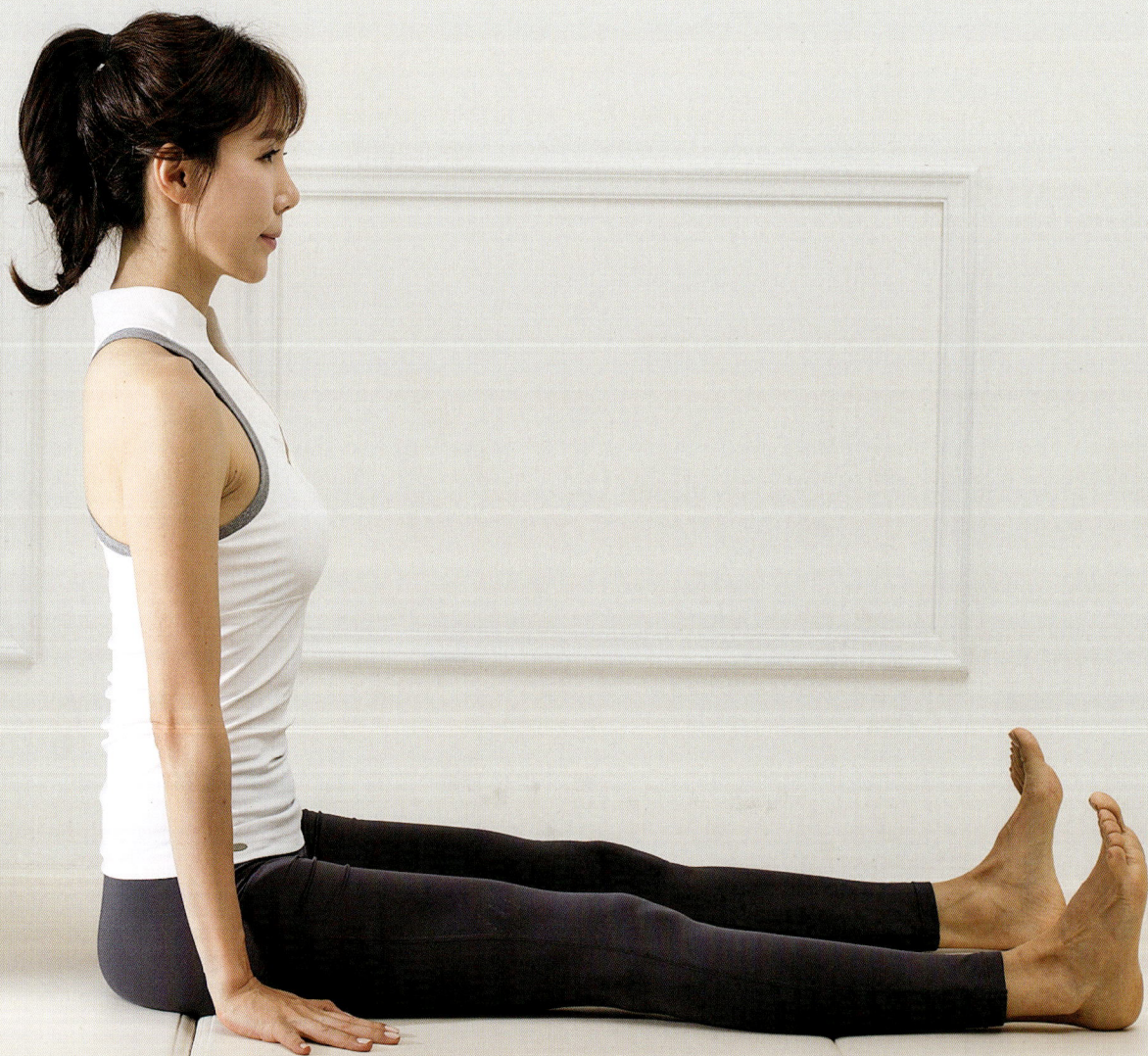

Neutral Posture

The sitting position, which requires sitting with your back straight, may be tough if you lack flexibility. Try to sit with both legs stretched out, but if you can't, bend your knees a little and try to keep your back straight. Since it's easier to sit straight when your legs are spread apart, you can also widen your leg position to suit your flexibility while maintaining good posture.

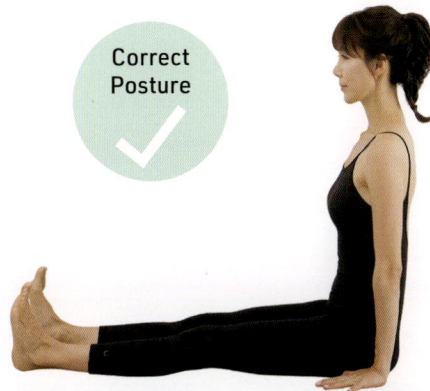

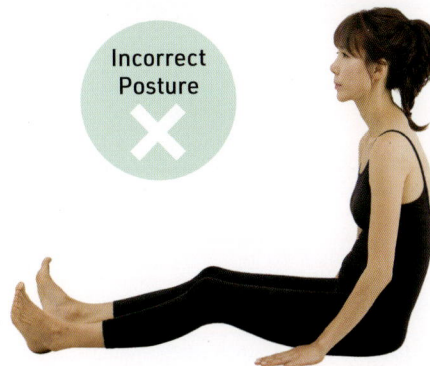

Correct Posture ✓

Incorrect Posture ✗

Spine Stretch Forward

This exercise can relax the back and strengthen overall muscles throughout the body, focusing on the spine and pelvis.

Sitting 1

1 Sit with your spine straightened, legs shoulder-width apart, and flex your feet.

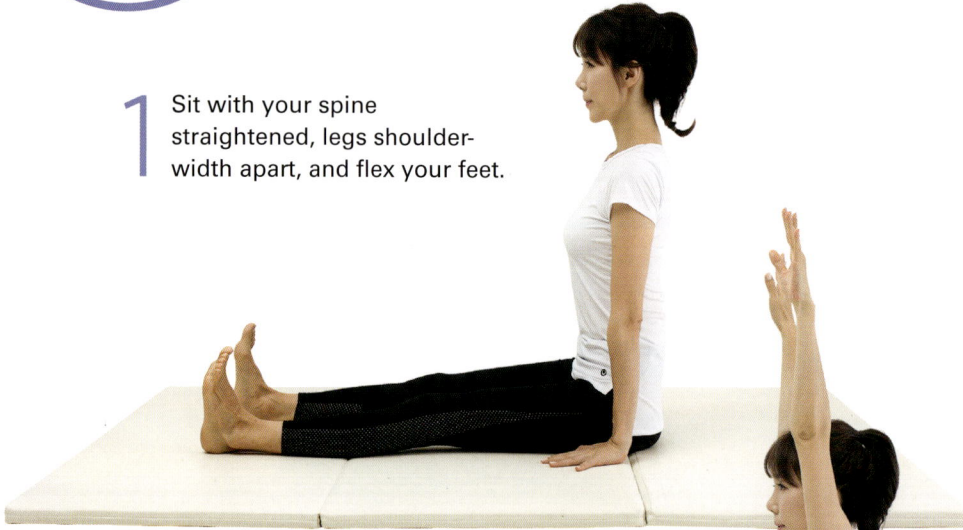

2 Raise both arms while straightening your spine as you inhale.

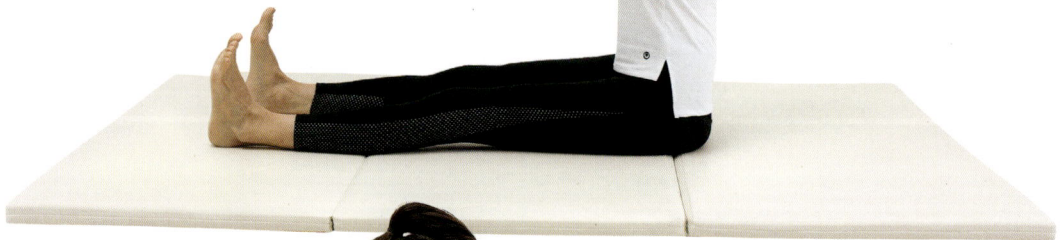

3 Lower your torso forward as you exhale.

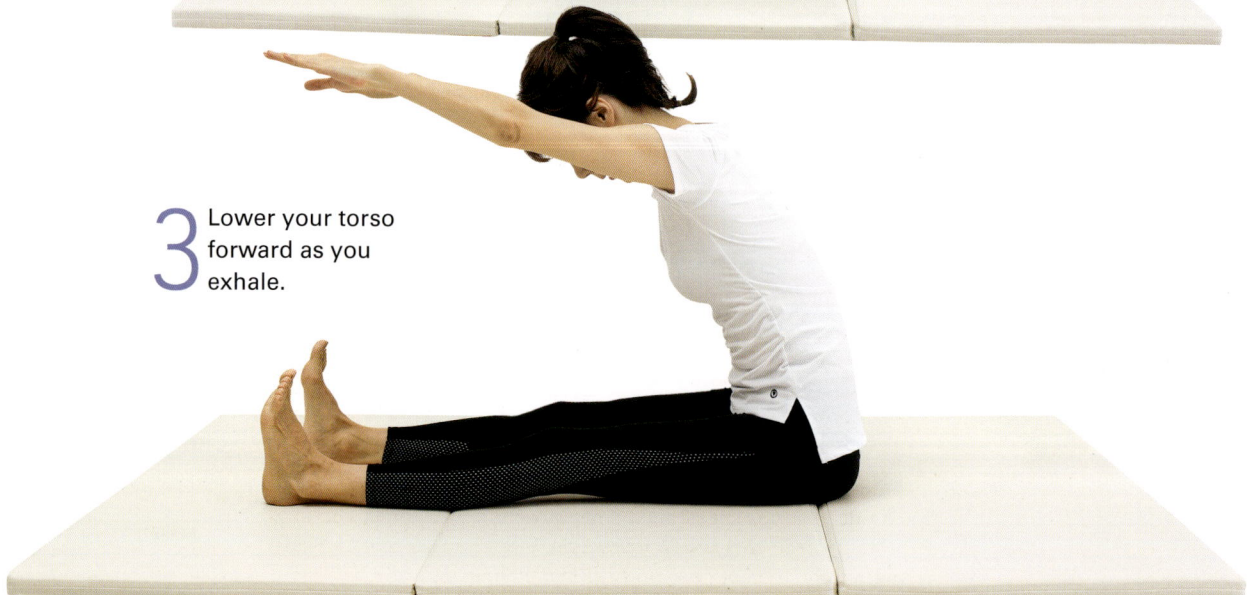

28

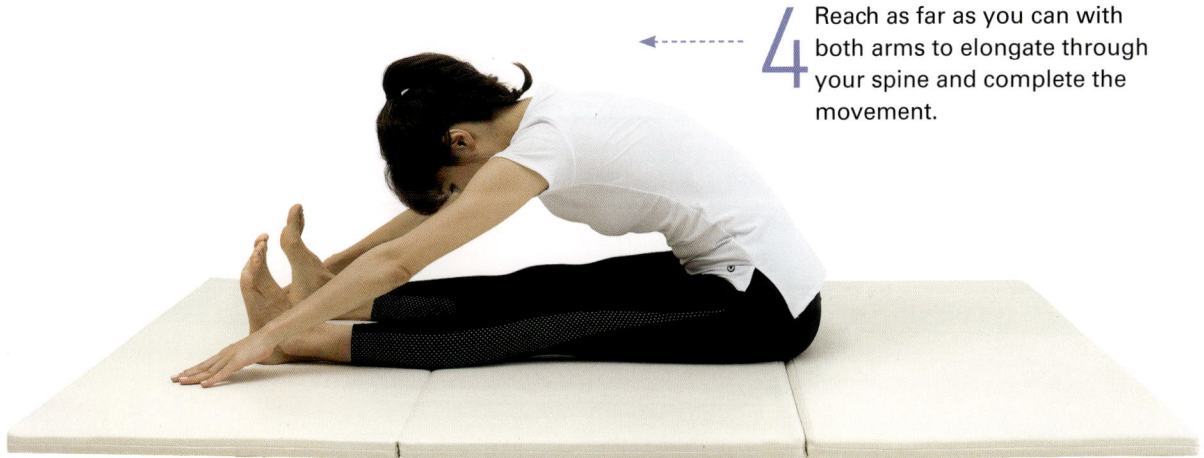

4 Reach as far as you can with both arms to elongate through your spine and complete the movement.

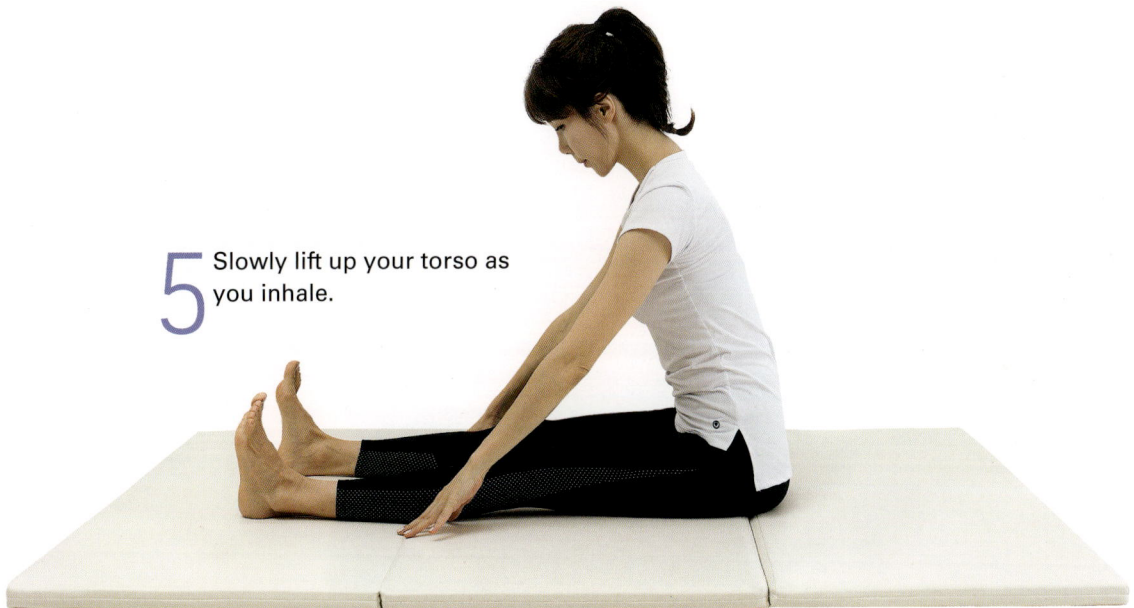

5 Slowly lift up your torso as you inhale.

* Repeat movements 4 and 5 three times for three sets.

Tip

When lowering your torso, try to move your body forward rather than bending your back. Do not lower your head too much. If your knees bend when lowering your torso, you may not get the best result. If possible, keep the back of your knees touching the floor as you stretch your legs.

Sitting 2

Calf Stretch

This exercise can increase flexibility in legs and blood circulation in the lower body. It can reduce lower body obesity and release pain in back of the knees.

1 Sit with your legs wide apart and flex both feet.

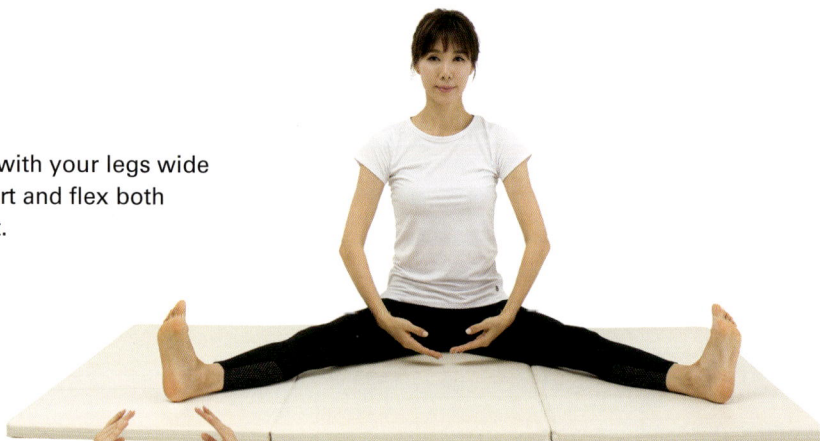

2 Raise your arms without tensing your shoulders to create an elegant posture.

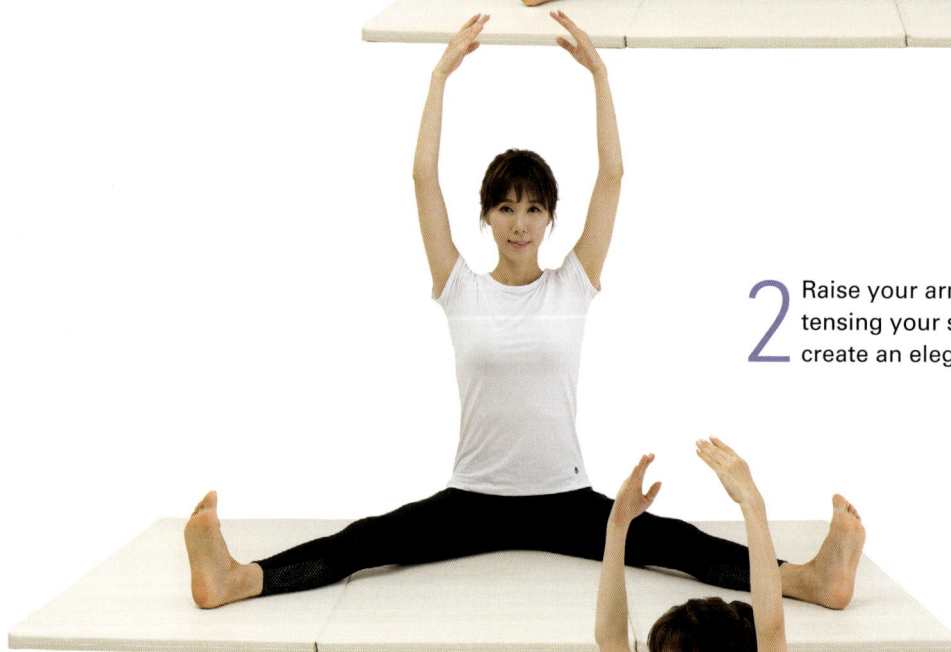

3 Inhale as you twist your torso to the right to set your starting position.

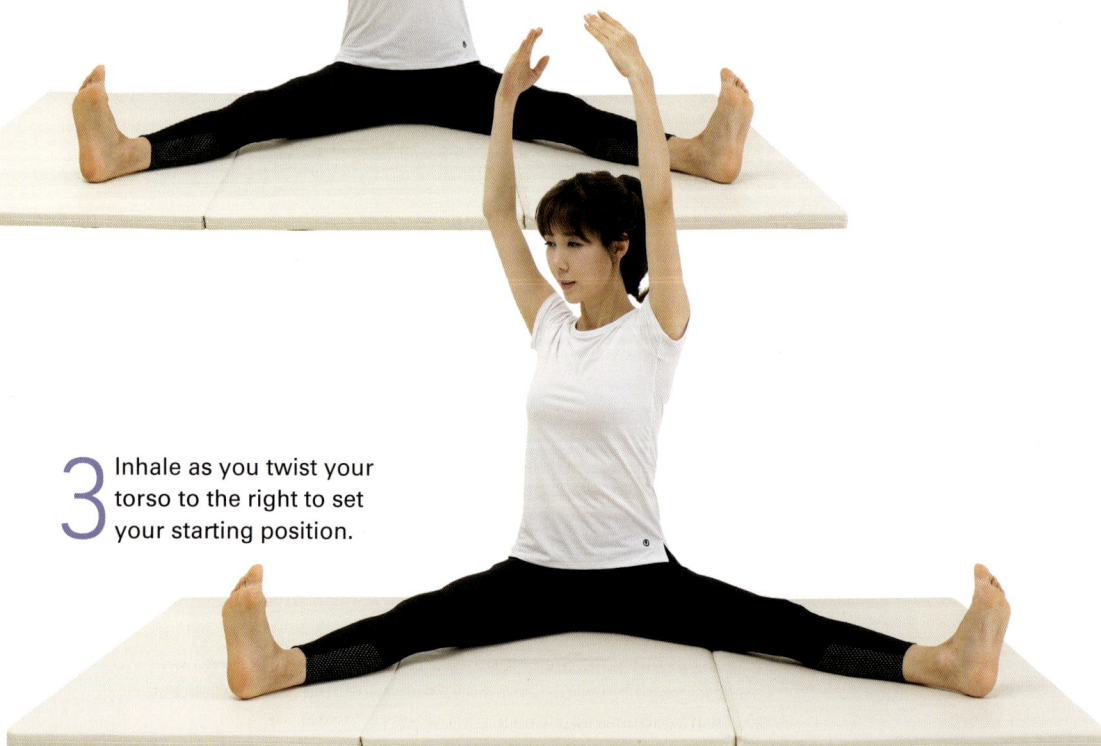

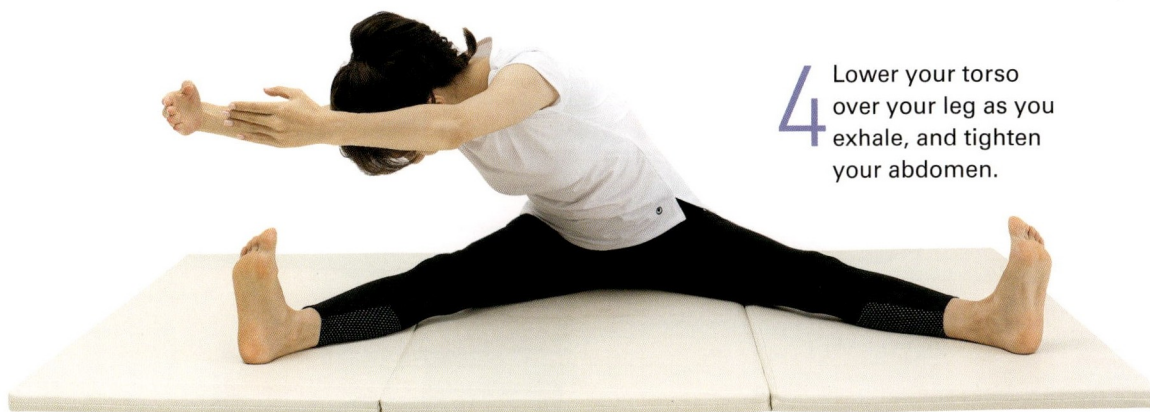

4 Lower your torso over your leg as you exhale, and tighten your abdomen.

* Repeat four times on each side.

Variation

Your can also practice the movement with one leg bent. Twist to the right with your left leg bent, and twist to the left with your right leg bent. Repeat four times on each leg.

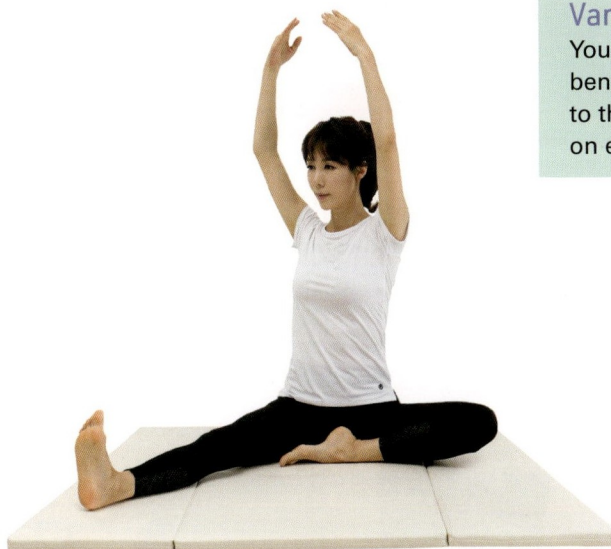

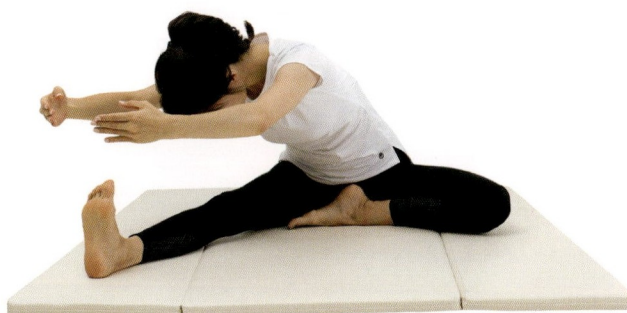

Tip

When flexing your feet, you need to stretch your legs without bending your knees and contract your leg muscles tight enough to make your heels almost rise off the floor.

The Saw

Improve flexibility and lower-body strength by twisting the torso and engaging Pilates breathing.

1 Spread your legs wider than your shoulder and reach both arms to the sides.

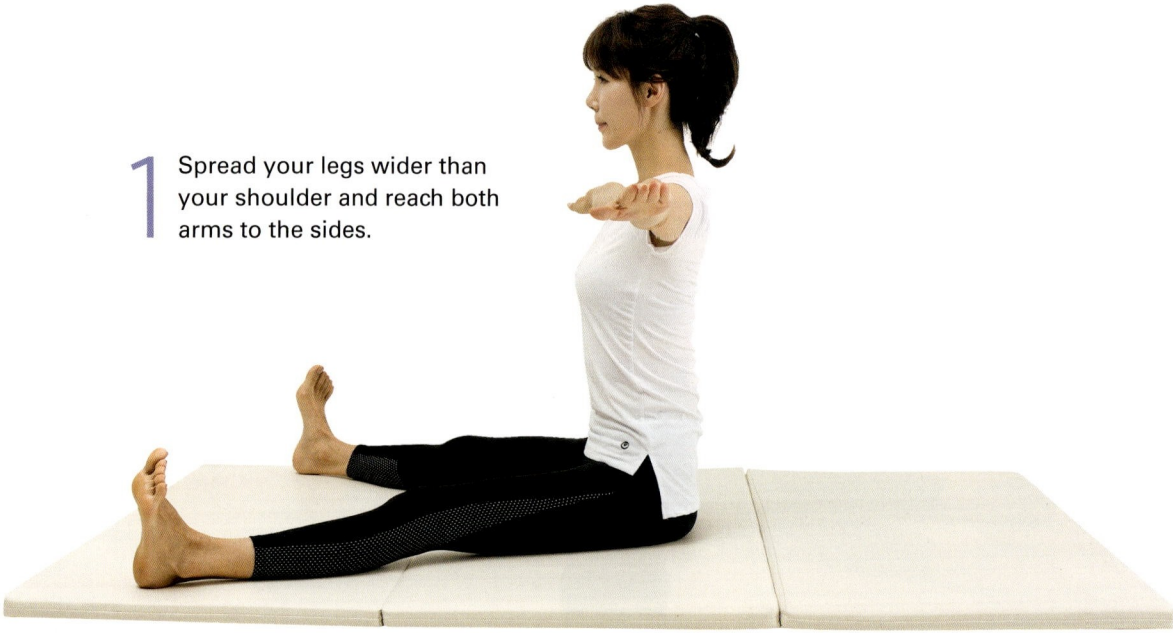

2 Twist your torso as you inhale, bringing the left arm backward and the right arm forward.

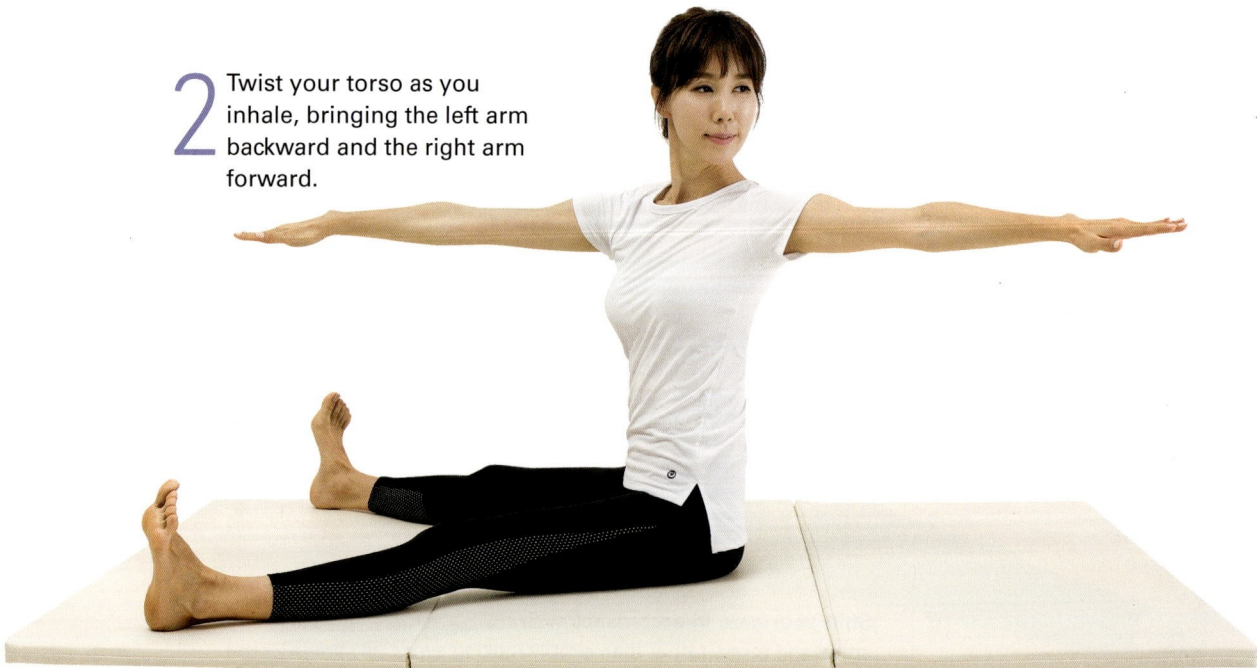

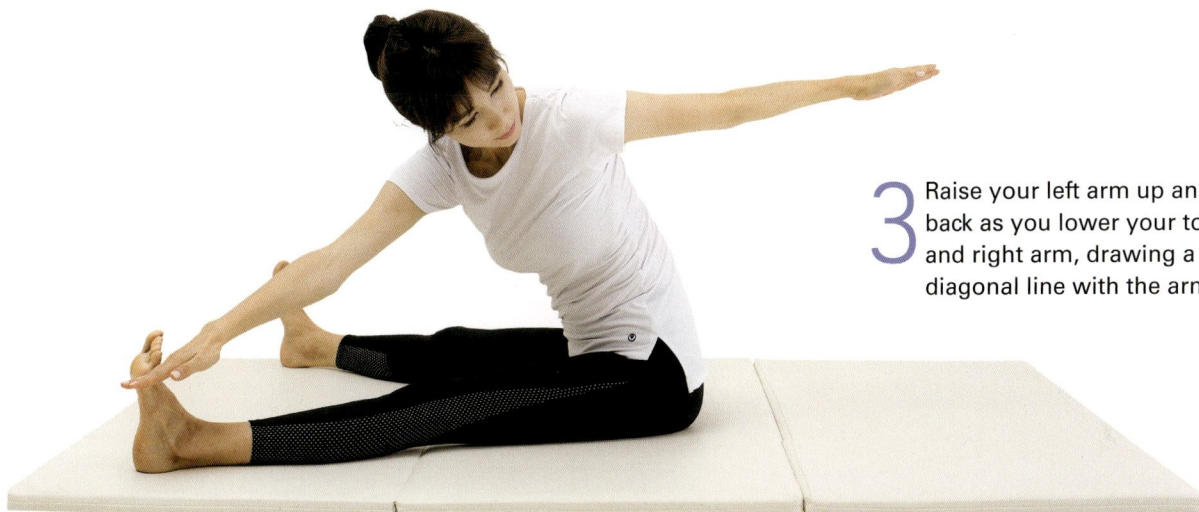

3 Raise your left arm up and back as you lower your torso and right arm, drawing a diagonal line with the arms.

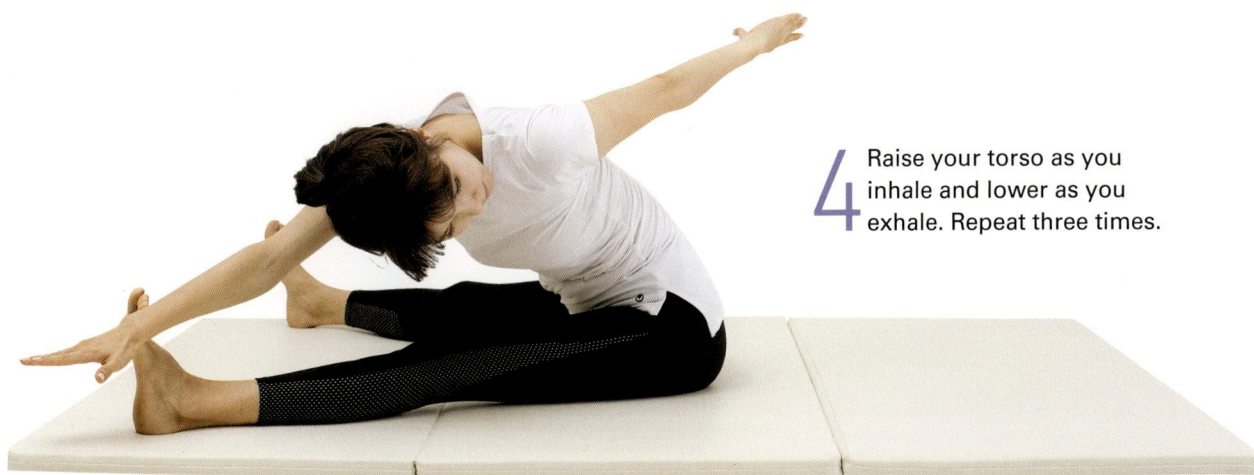

4 Raise your torso as you inhale and lower as you exhale. Repeat three times.

* Repeat two sets of movement 4 on each side.

--- Tip ---

As you twist and reach forward, your lower arm should lightly touch the outside of the opposite foot, as if sawing. Raise your arms backward as high as you can and deeply lower your torso as you exhale.

Sitting

5

The Teaser

This exercise is a classic Pilates position that strengthens abdominal muscles and improves balance and focus.

1 Sit with your knees bent and lift your heels off the floor.

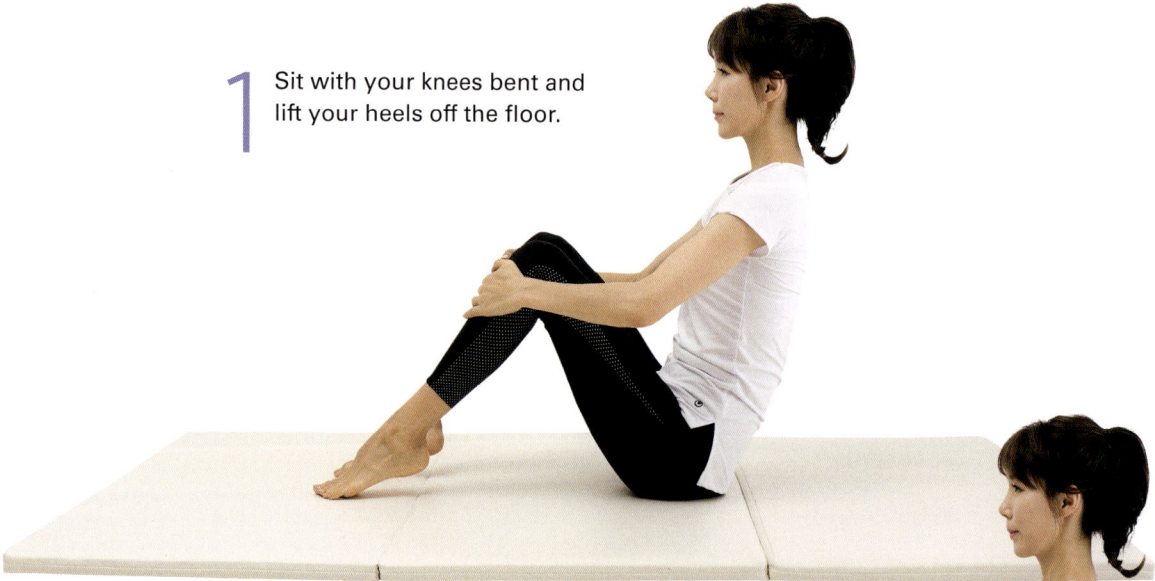

2 Lift up both legs, maintaining your balance.

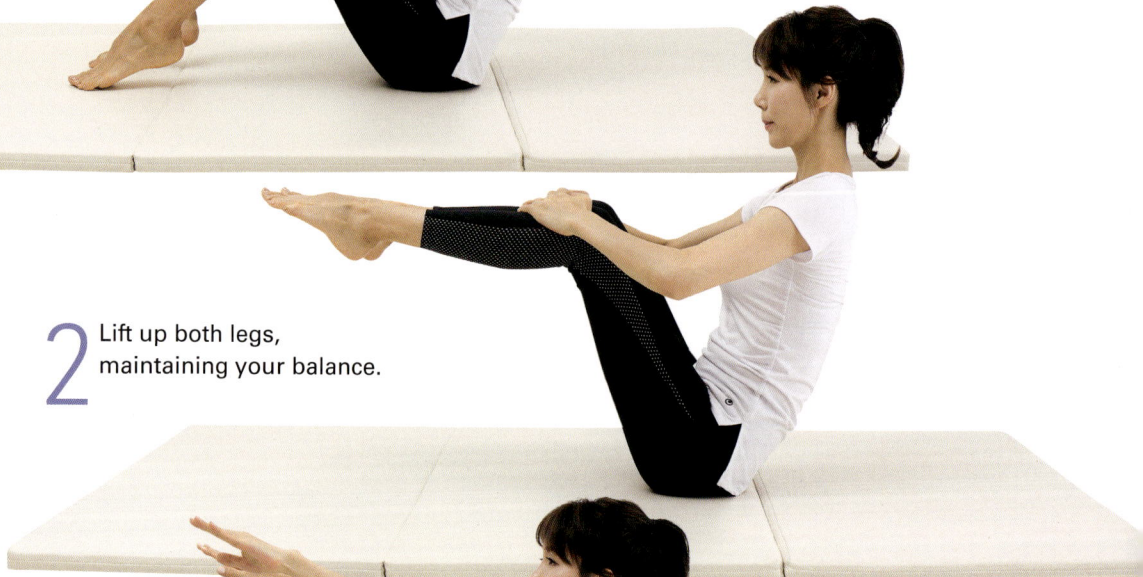

3 Stretch both arms forward while keeping your posture still.

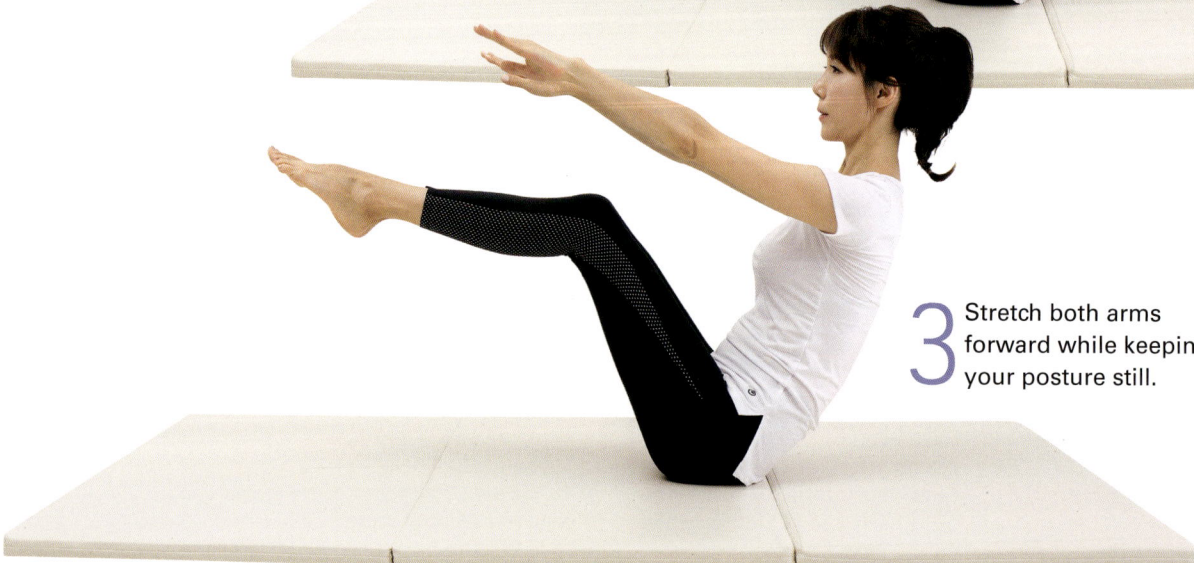

4 Make your legs parallel with the arms to complete the posture.

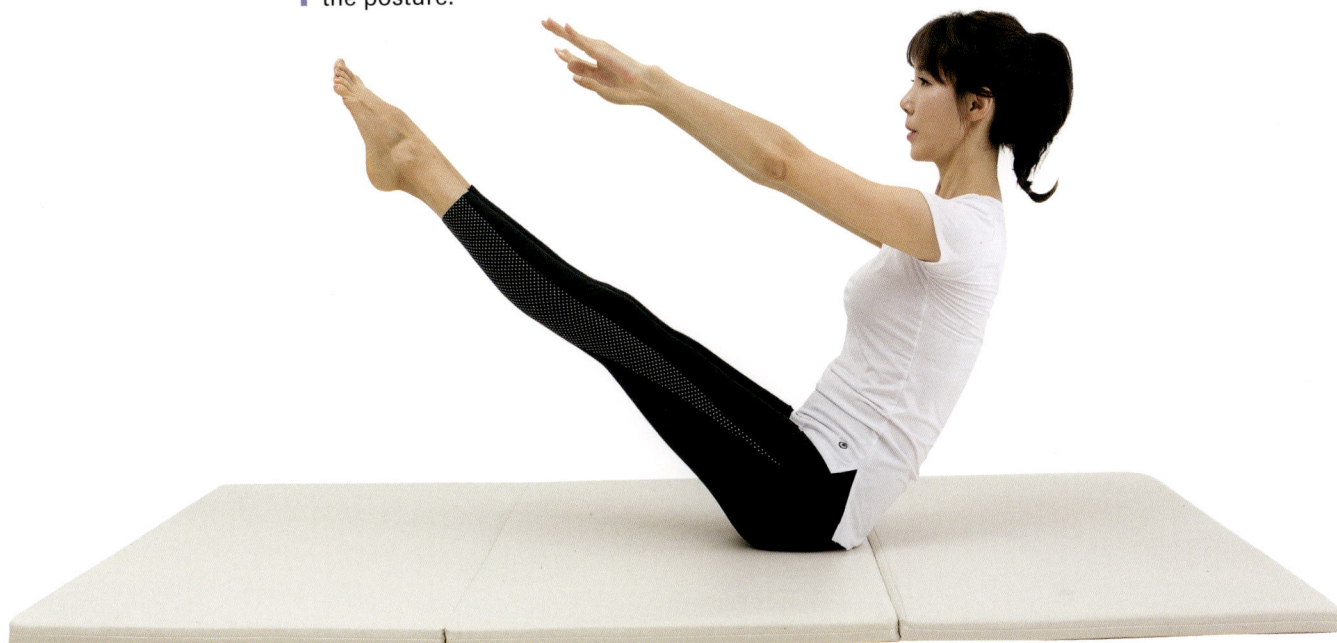

* Repeat three sets of movements 1 to 4.

Tip

When you become more familiar with the movement, practice starting from the supine position instead of the sitting position.

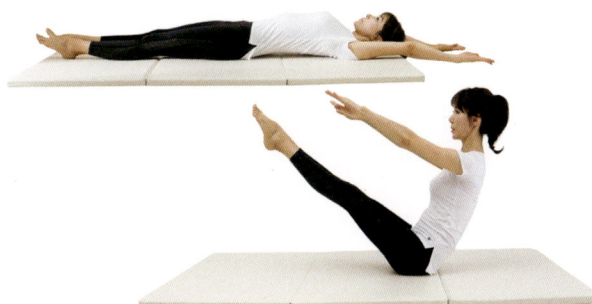

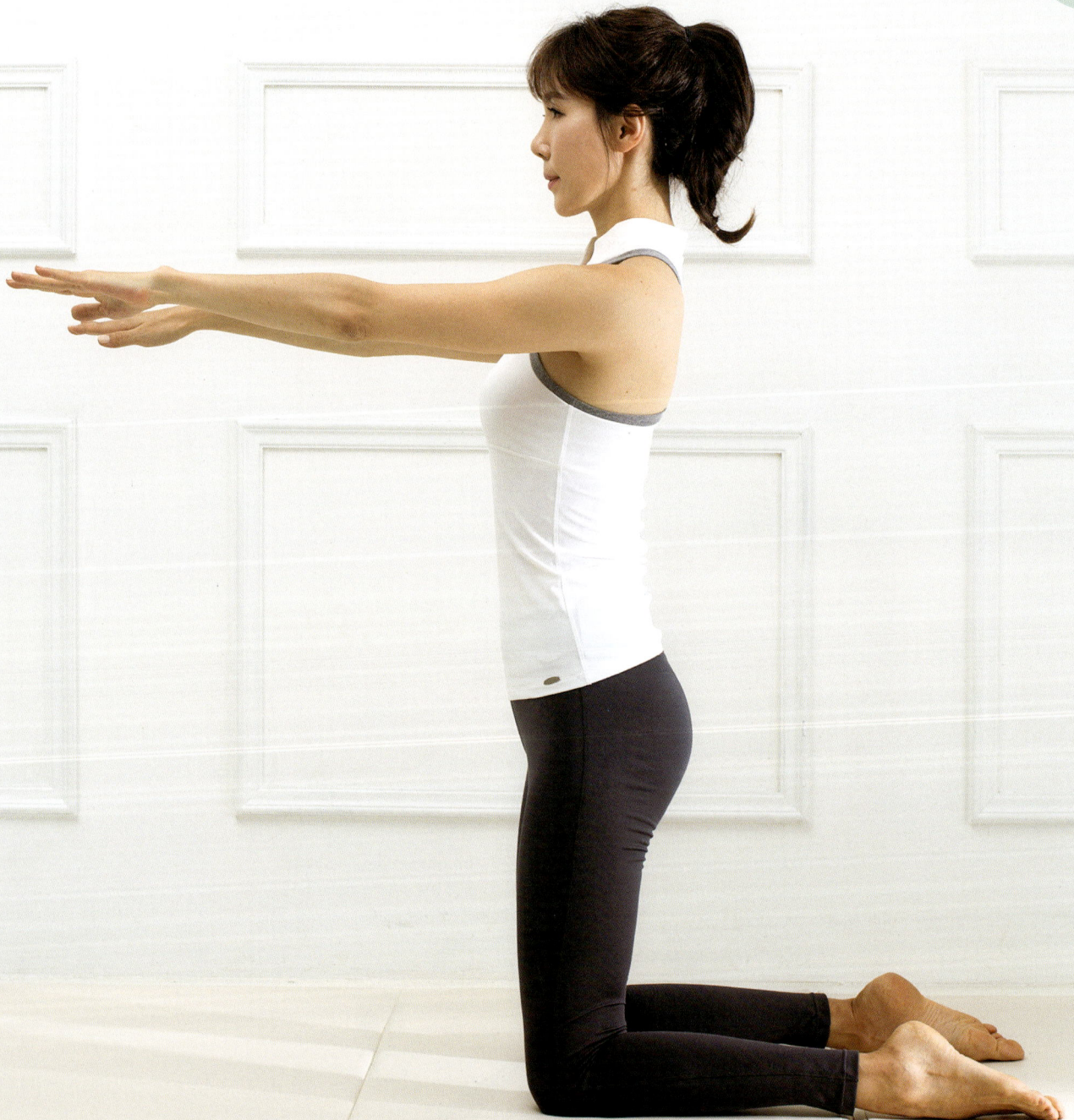

Neutral Posture

The kneeling position can be challenging, as it requires balance and flexibility. When practicing an unfamiliar posture, notice how your body changes as you wake up underutilized muscles. Try not to overtighten the muscles, as this will cause unnecessary arching of the chest and back. Also, be conscious of your core so that your stomach doesn't stick out and you maintain the natural curve of the spine.

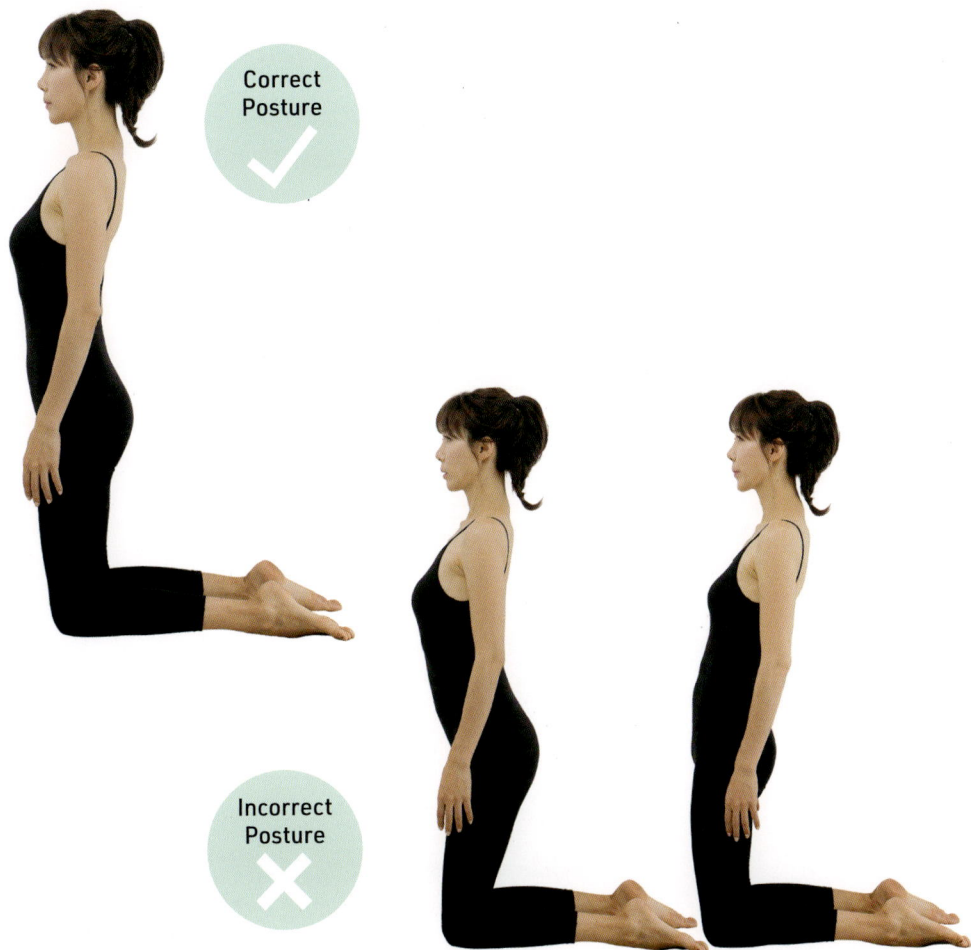

Correct Posture ✓

Incorrect Posture ✗

Thigh Stretching
Improve flexibility and sculpt your lower body by toning your core, glutes, and thighs.

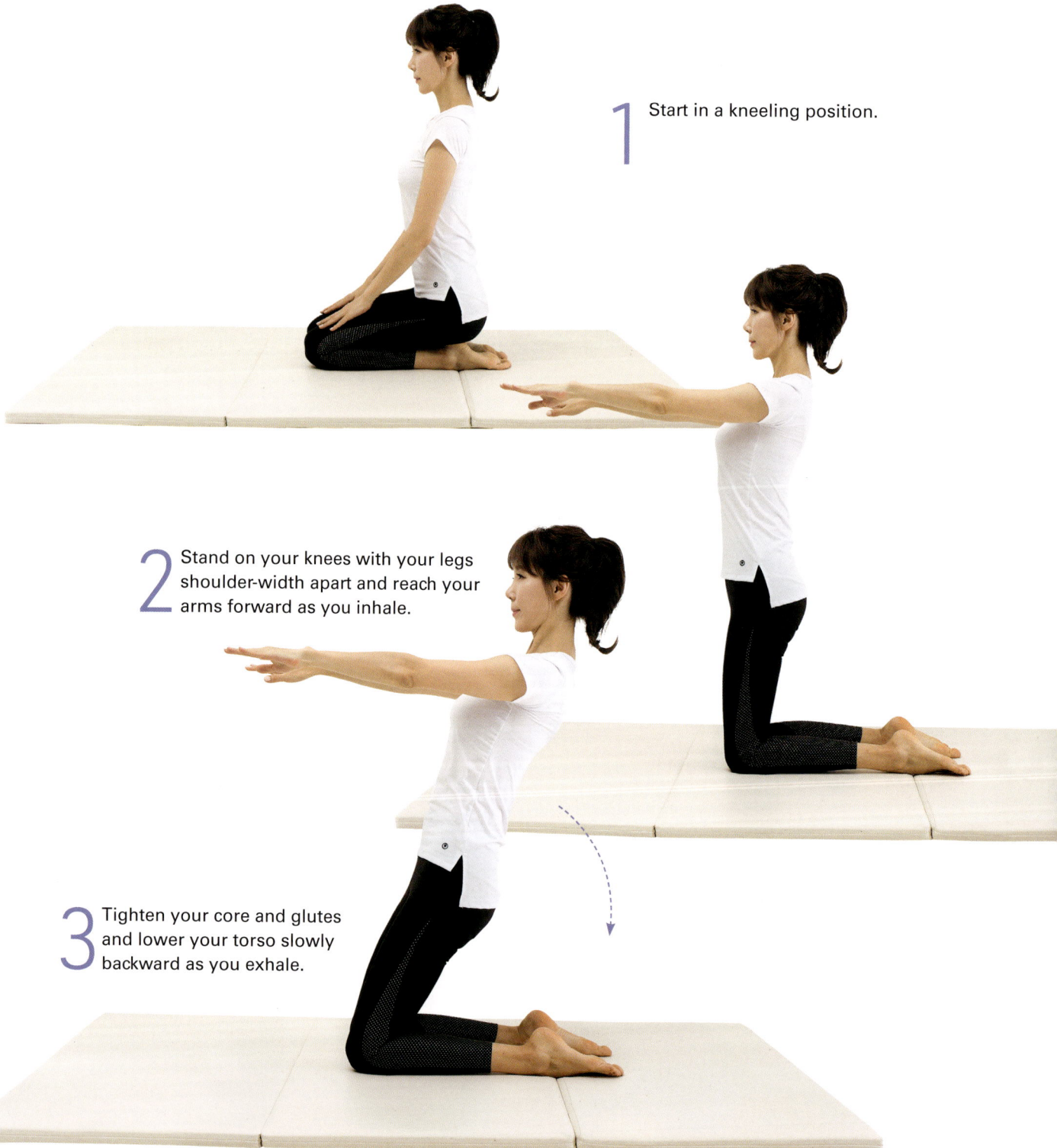

1 Start in a kneeling position.

2 Stand on your knees with your legs shoulder-width apart and reach your arms forward as you inhale.

3 Tighten your core and glutes and lower your torso slowly backward as you exhale.

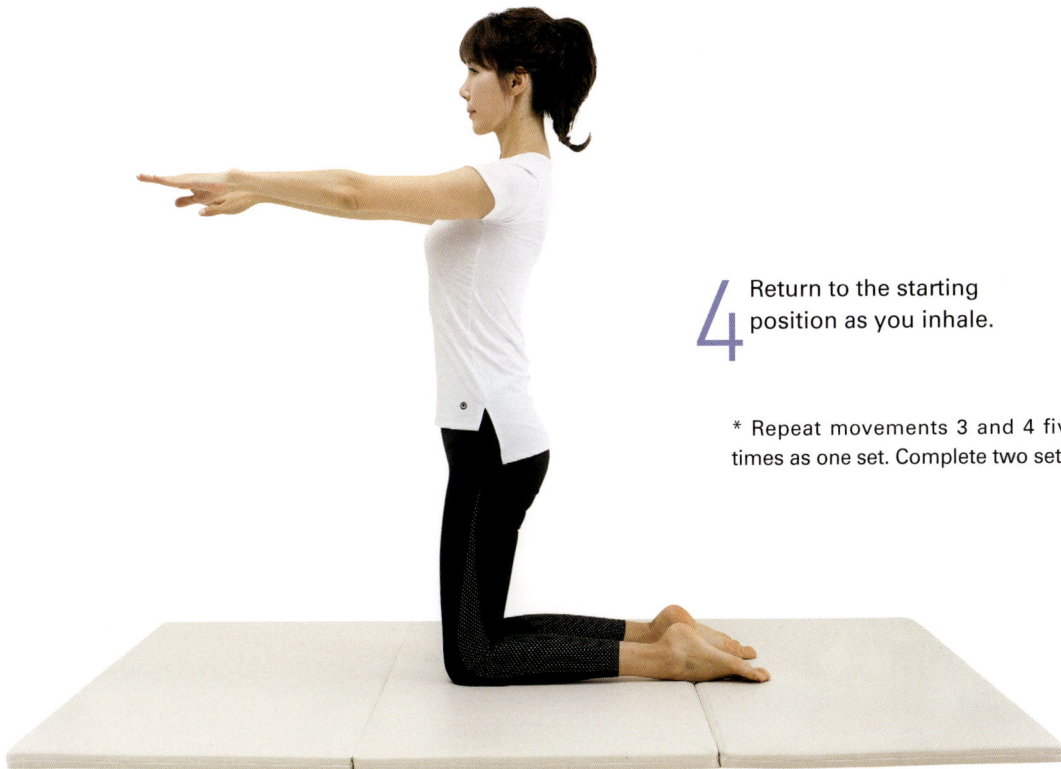

4 Return to the starting position as you inhale.

* Repeat movements 3 and 4 five times as one set. Complete two sets.

--- Tip ---

If you lack abdominal strength or overdo the movement, you may injure yourself as your legs weaken. Be careful not to work out beyond your capability by keeping the movement within the range of your muscle mobility.

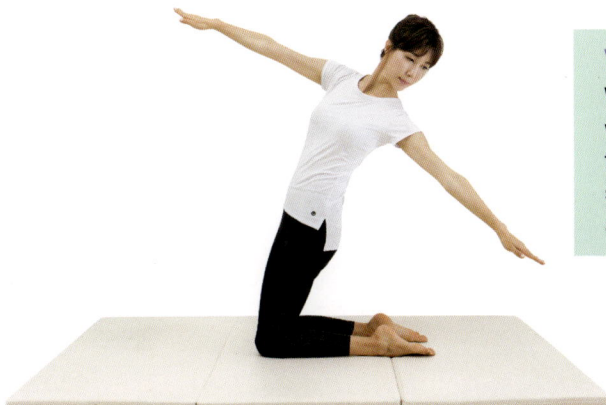

Variation
When you become familiar with the movement, try twisting your body to each side with your arms extended as you lower your torso.

Kneeling Squat

Similar to a regular standing squat, the kneeling version is easier to perform. It will strengthen your erector spinae and gluteal muscles.

1 Sit with your knees pelvis-width apart with both hands placed behind your head as you inhale.

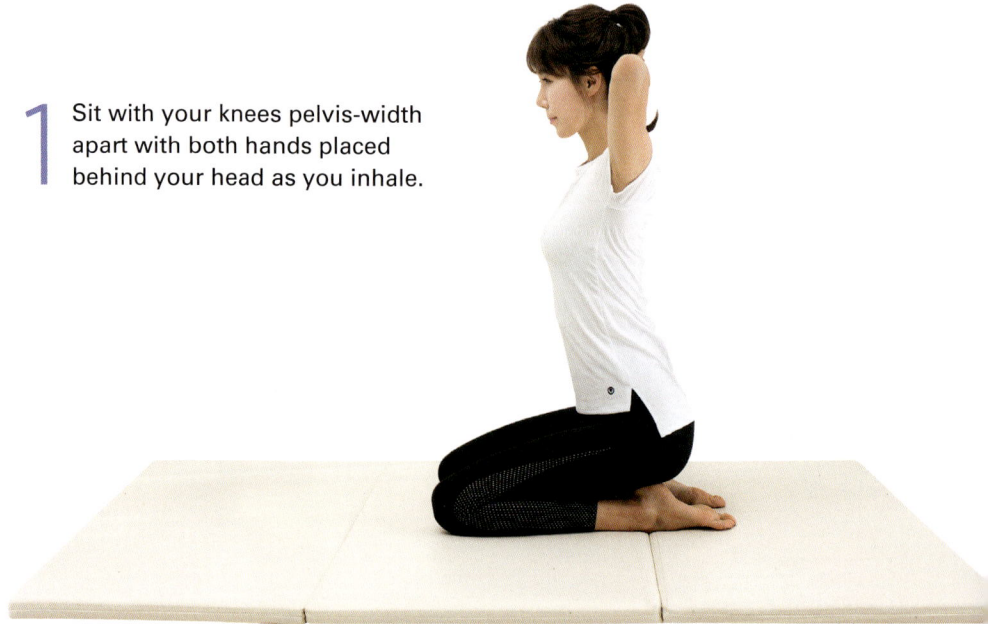

2 Rise up straight with your torso and engage your hip muscles as you exhale.

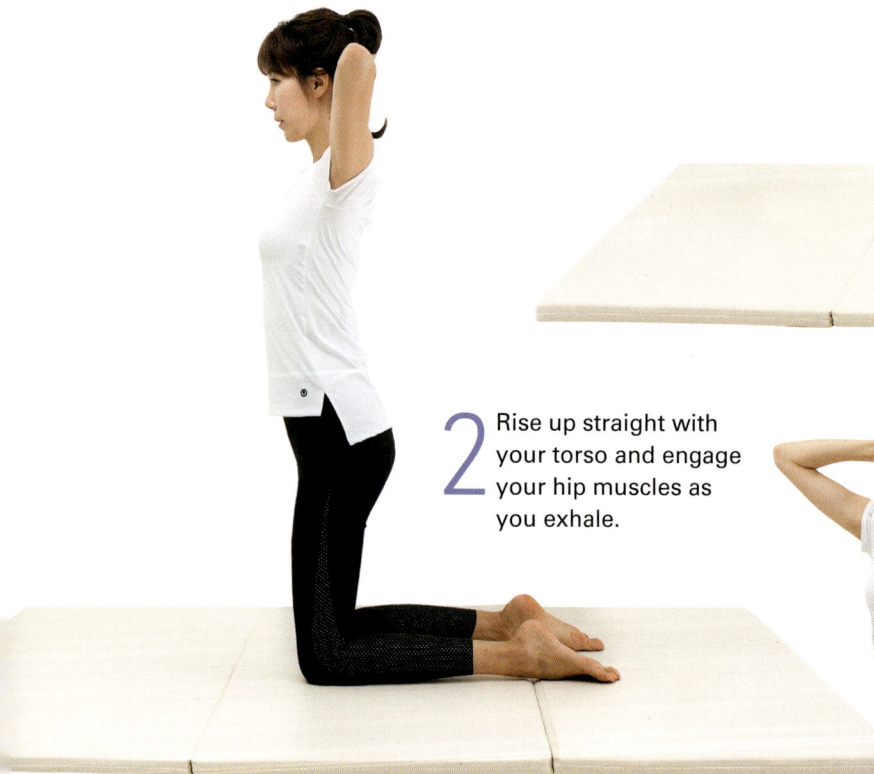

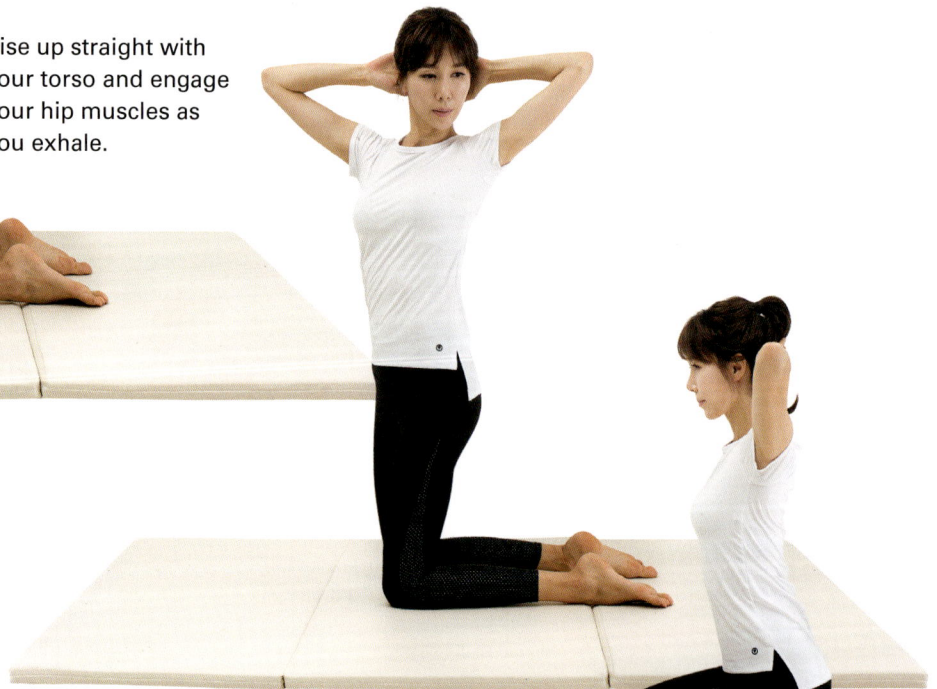

3 Twist your torso to the left, then return to the starting position, kneeling down.

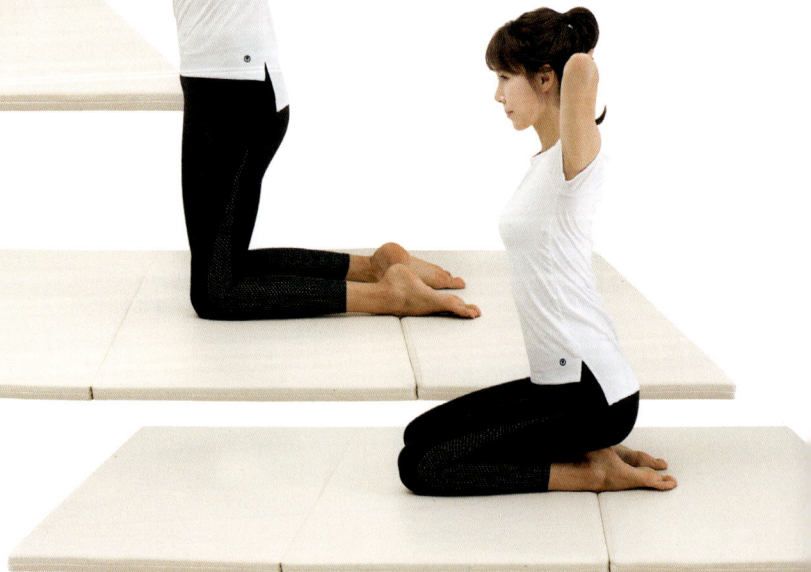

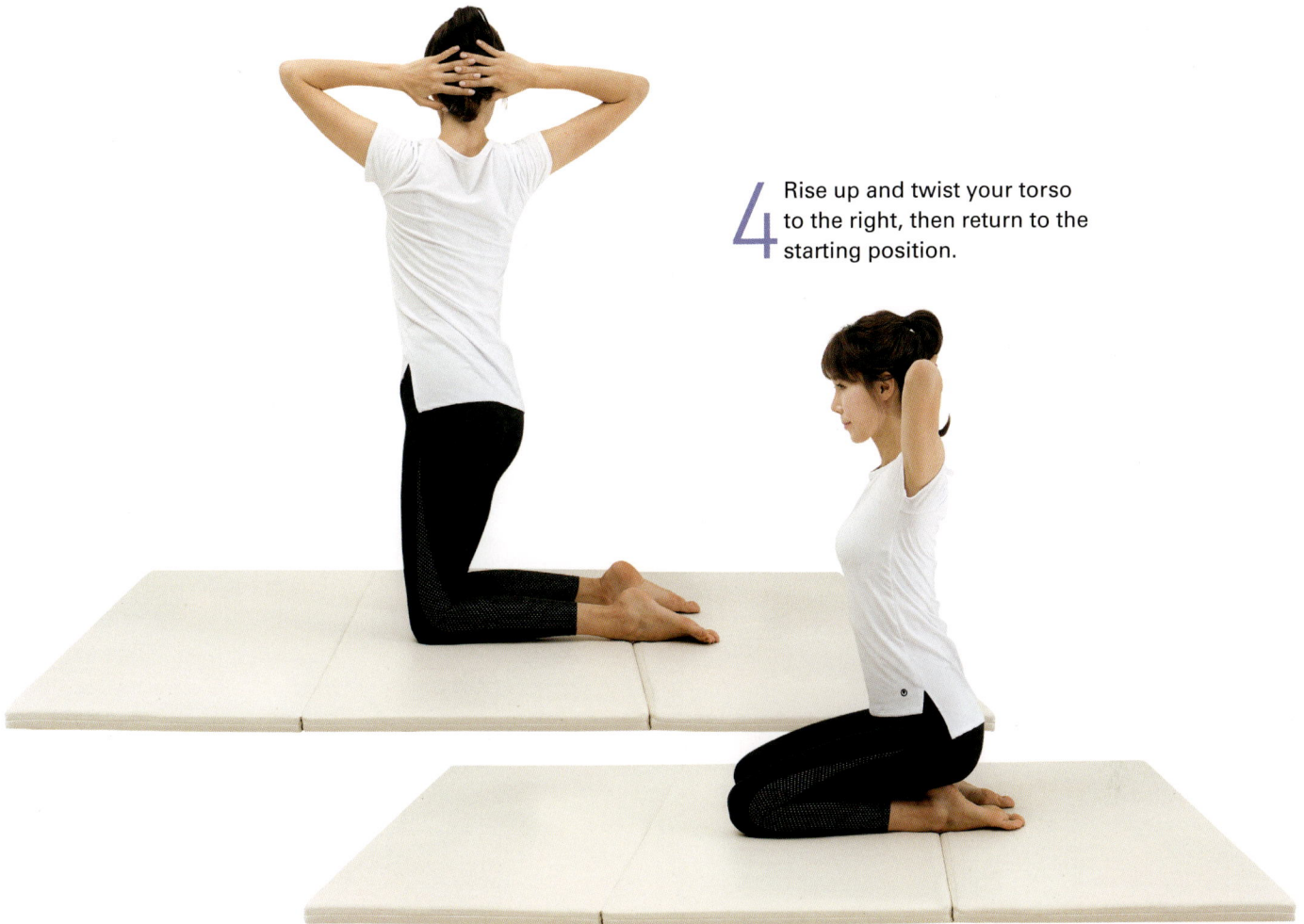

4 Rise up and twist your torso to the right, then return to the starting position.

* Rise up and twist your torso to the right, then sit down; rise up and twist your torso to the left, then sit down. Repeat this movement 10 times on each side.

— Tip —

To maintain the correct alignment of the spine, it's important to train the core muscles. Practice the movements regularly, focusing on the abdominal, back, gluteal, and thigh muscles.

Kneeling Side-Leg Lift

This exercise will improve balance and tone your lower body and glutes. It can also strengthen the hip joints.

1 Kneel down.

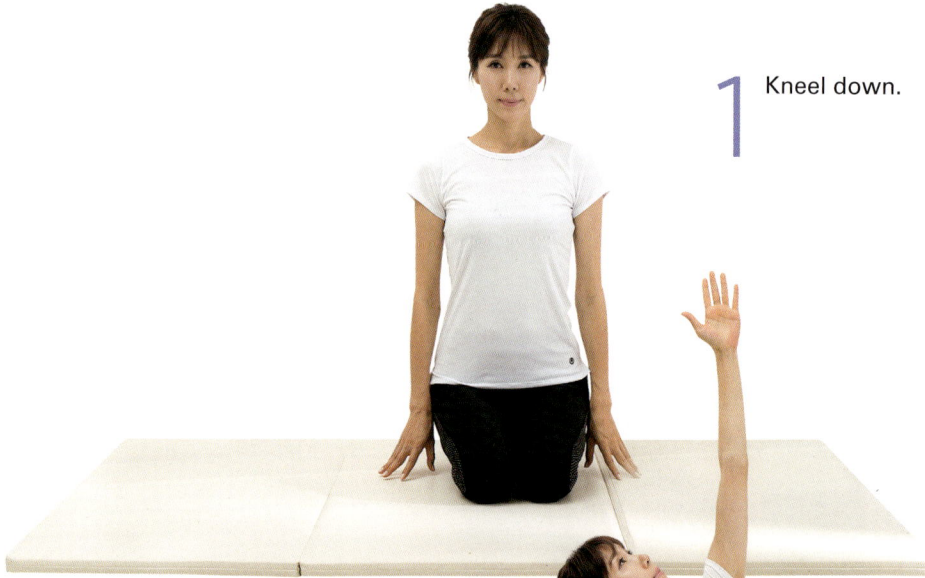

2 Place your right hand on the floor and stretch your left arm upward.

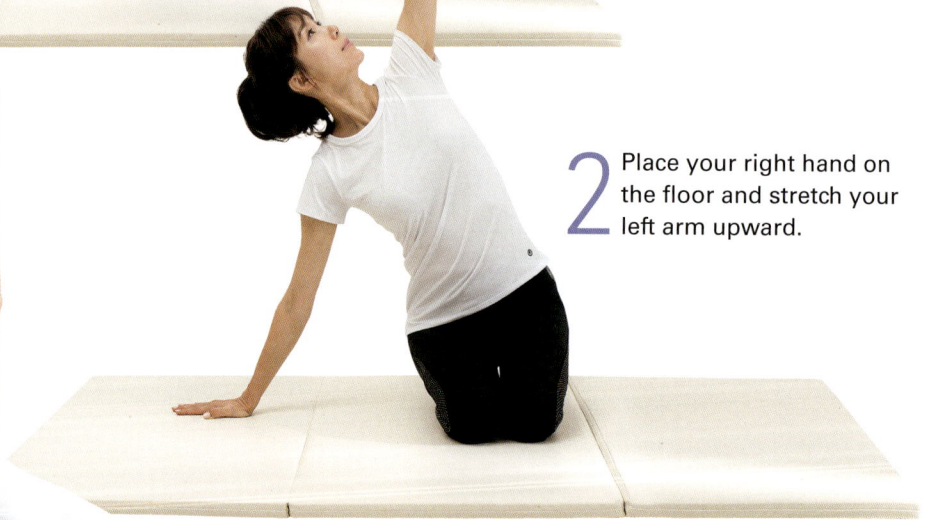

3 Lift up your torso as you inhale and stretch your left leg to touch the floor with your toe.

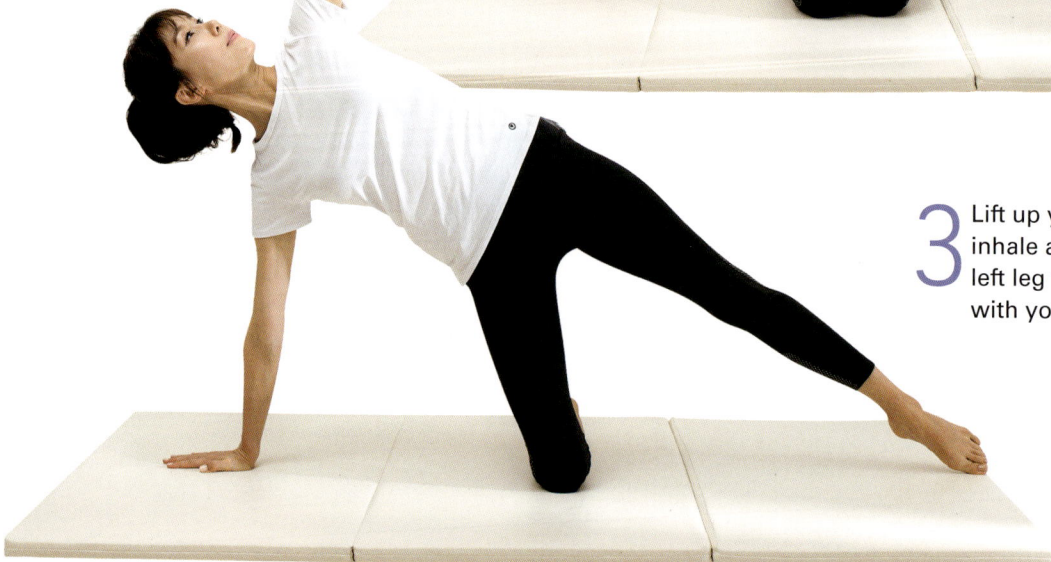

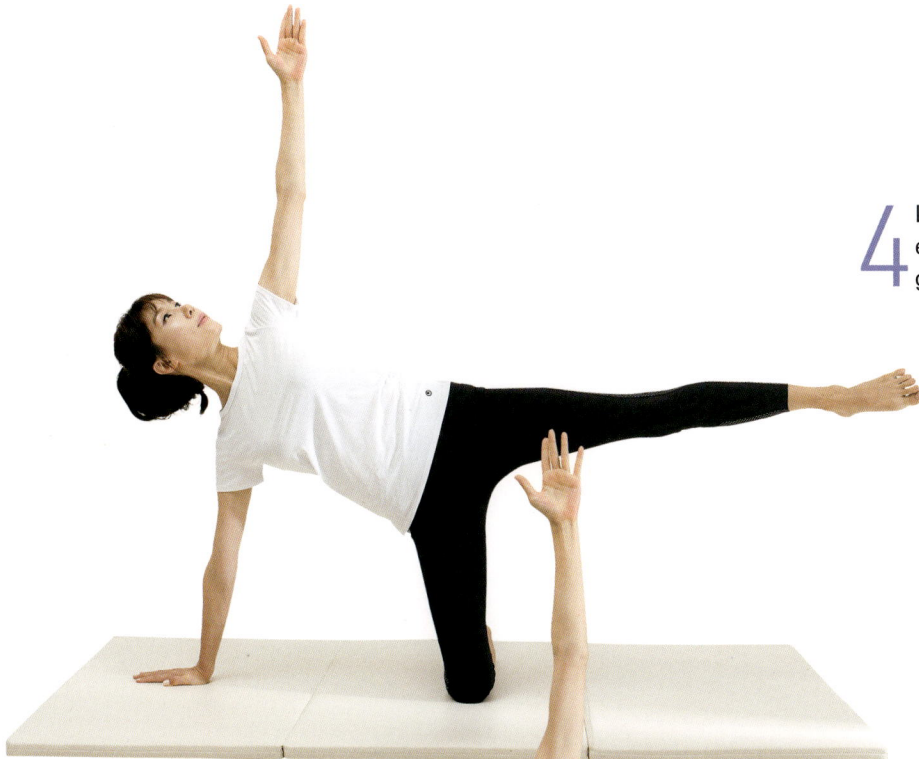

4 Lift your leg up as you exhale, while tightening the glutes.

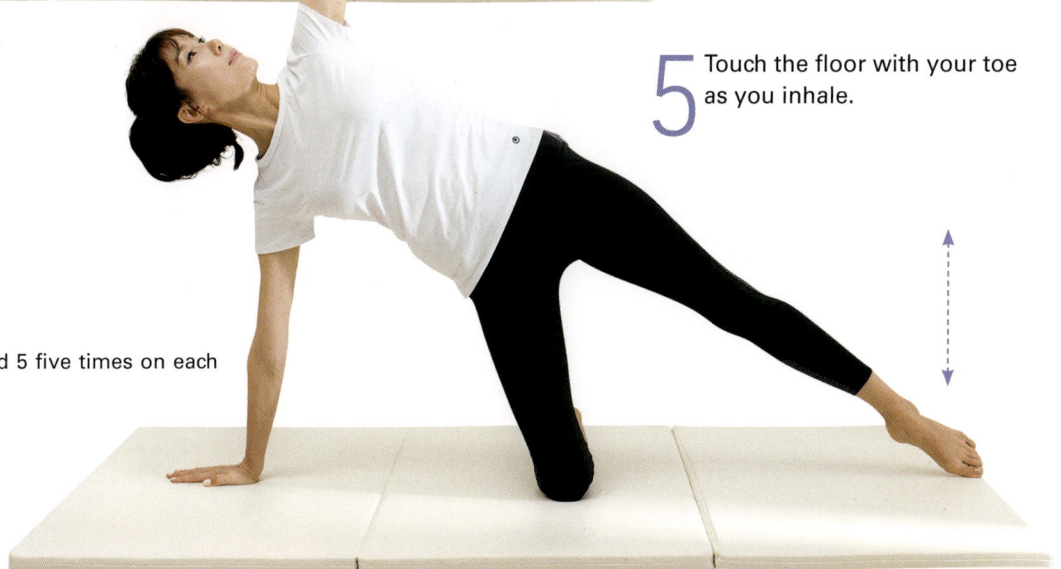

5 Touch the floor with your toe as you inhale.

* Repeat movements 4 and 5 five times on each side for two sets.

— Tip —

If your torso shakes, you might not get the desired results. Focus on controlling your body so you only move your legs.

Kneeling
4

Kneeling Side Bend

This exercise engages the sides of your body and increases flexibility and strength. It can also aid with digestion.

1 Kneel down.

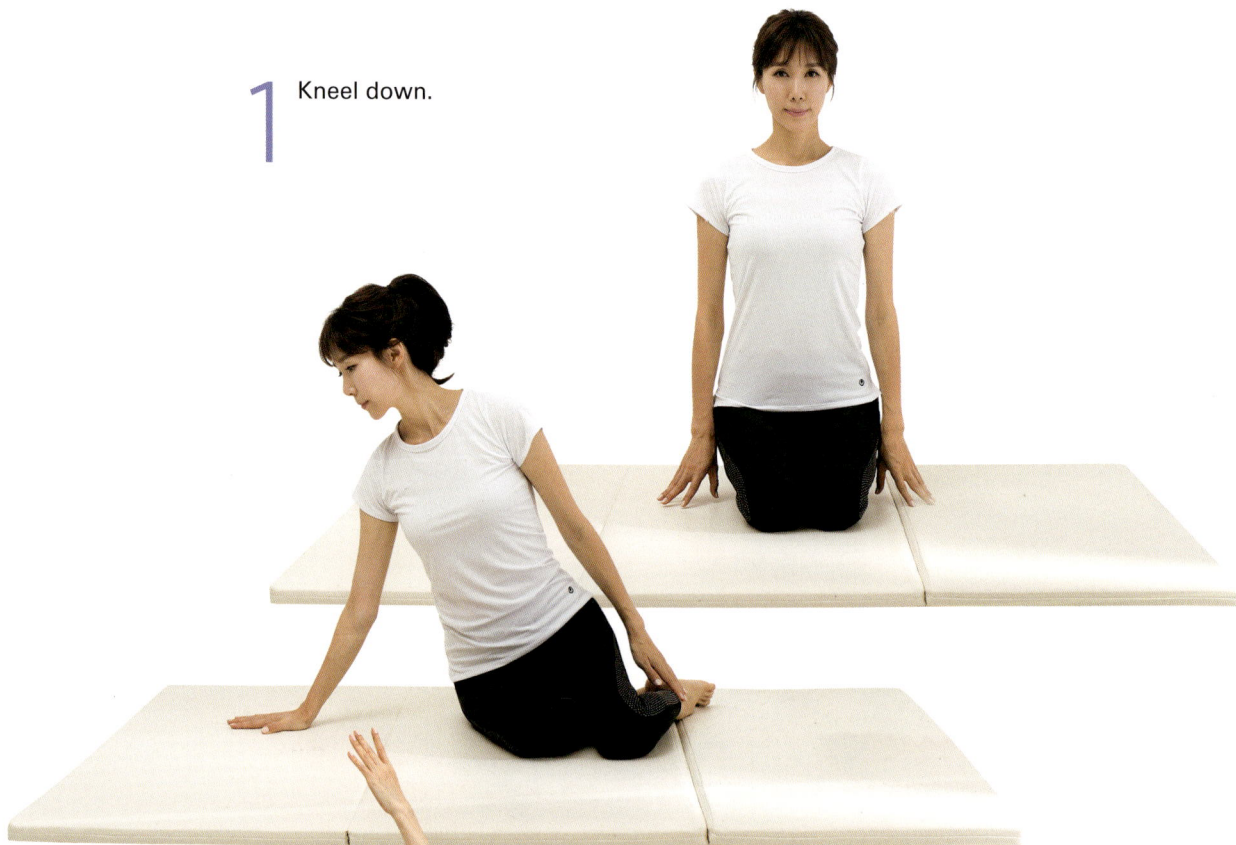

2 Place your right hand on the floor and lean your body to the right.

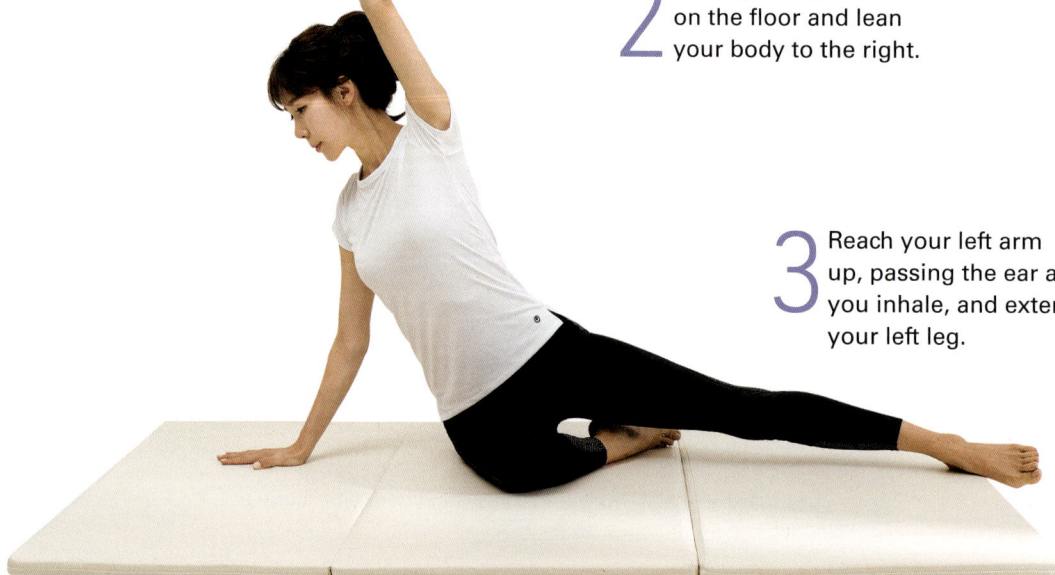

3 Reach your left arm up, passing the ear as you inhale, and extend your left leg.

4 Supporting with your right arm and right leg, lift your body up as you exhale.

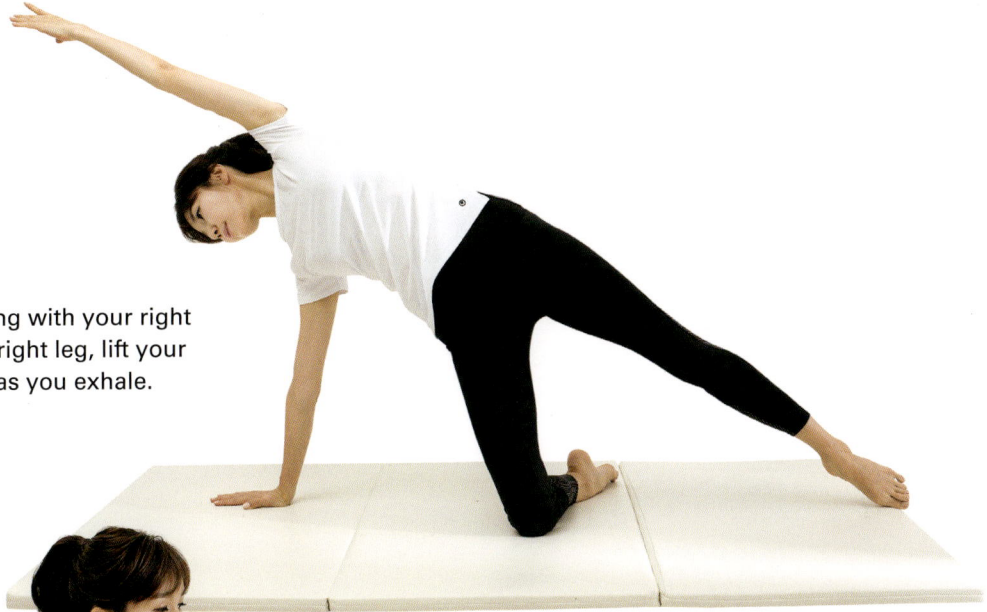

5 Lower your body and left arm as you inhale.

* Repeat movements 4 and 5 five times on each side for two sets.

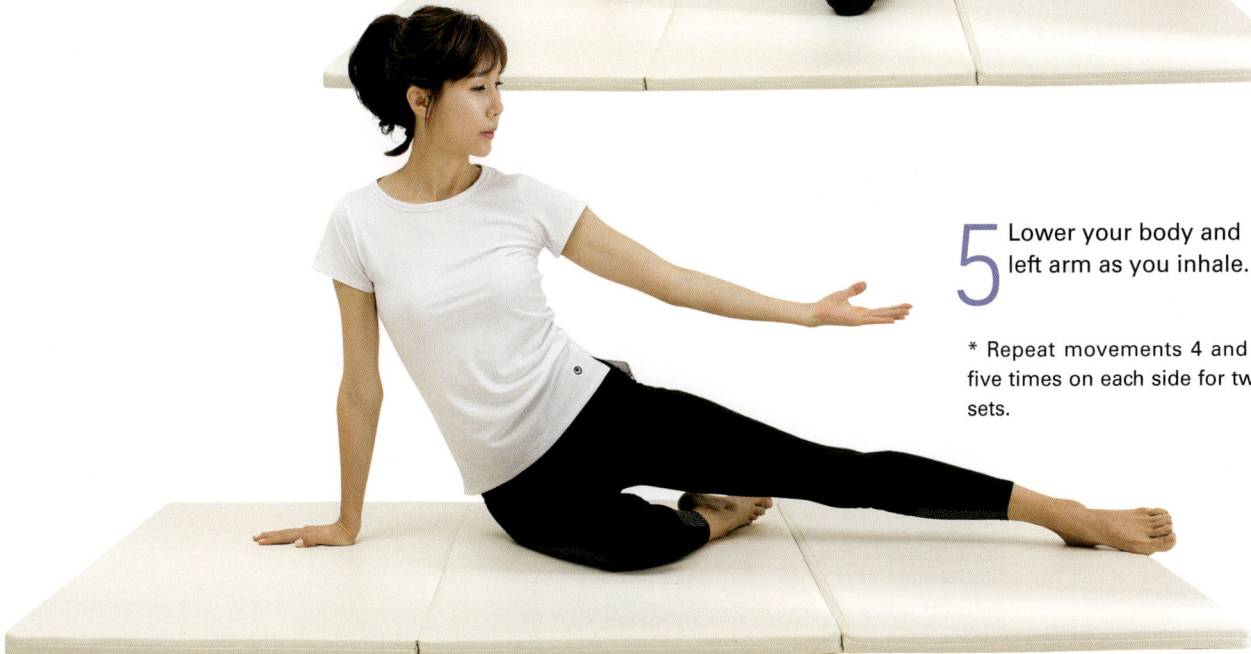

Tip

If you lift your torso too high, you can lose stability in your core, engaging only your arm. Stay mindful of your body's alignment as you exercise.

Side Lying

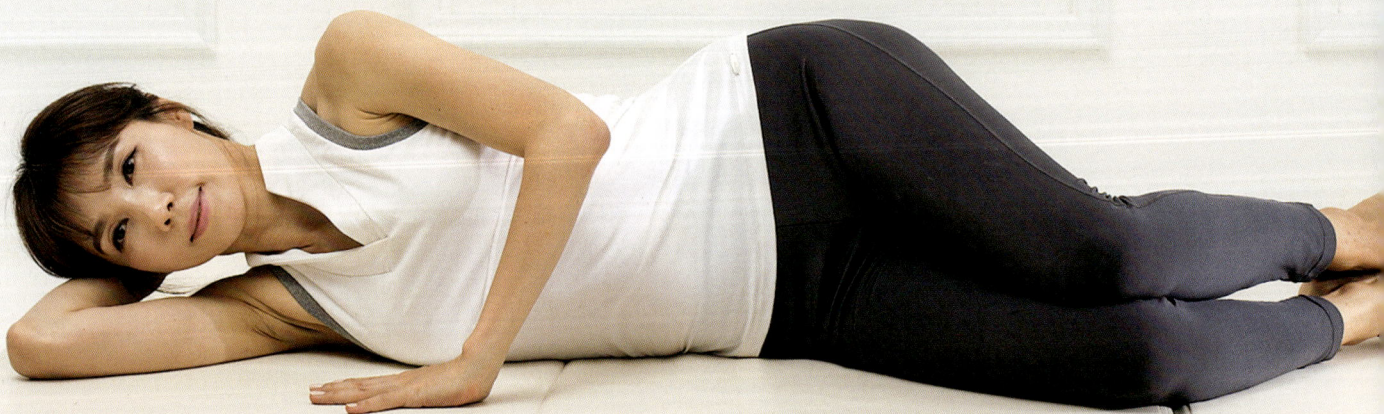

Neutral Posture

When lying on your side, support your head to keep your neck in a neutral position and prevent overbending. Always make sure to keep the side of your torso straight. Adjust your arms to make your neck comfortable and adjust the angle of your legs to balance.

Correct Posture ✓

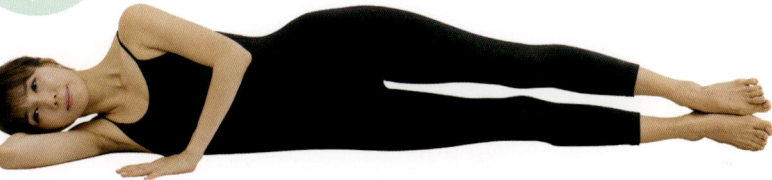

Incorrect Posture ✗

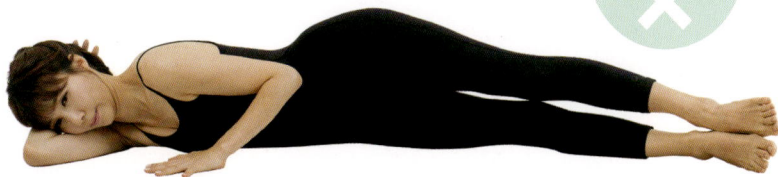

The Clam

This exercise strengthens the pelvis and gluteal muscles while helping to correct pelvis and leg misalignment.

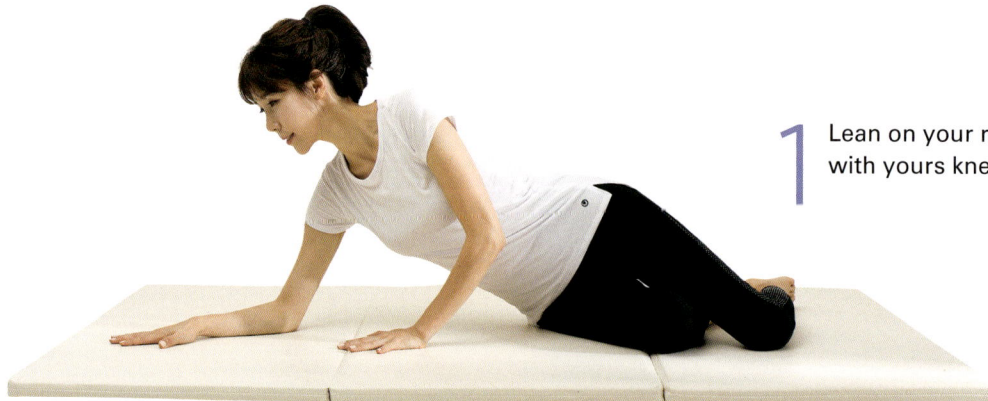

1 Lean on your right side with yours knees bent.

2 Lie on your right side with one arm supporting your head and tighten your core to align your spine.

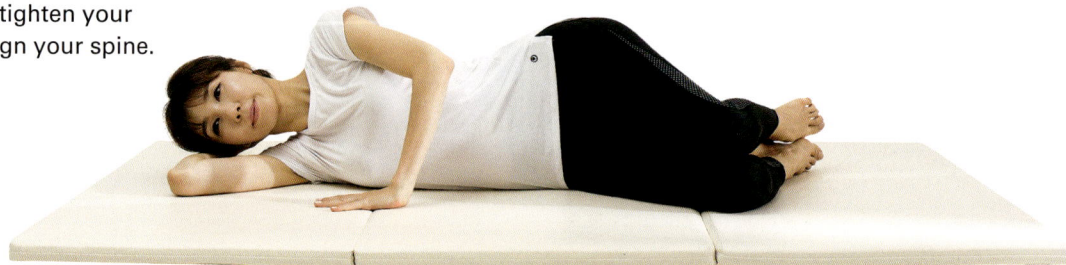

3 Tighten your core as you exhale, and contract your glutes while opening your left knee.

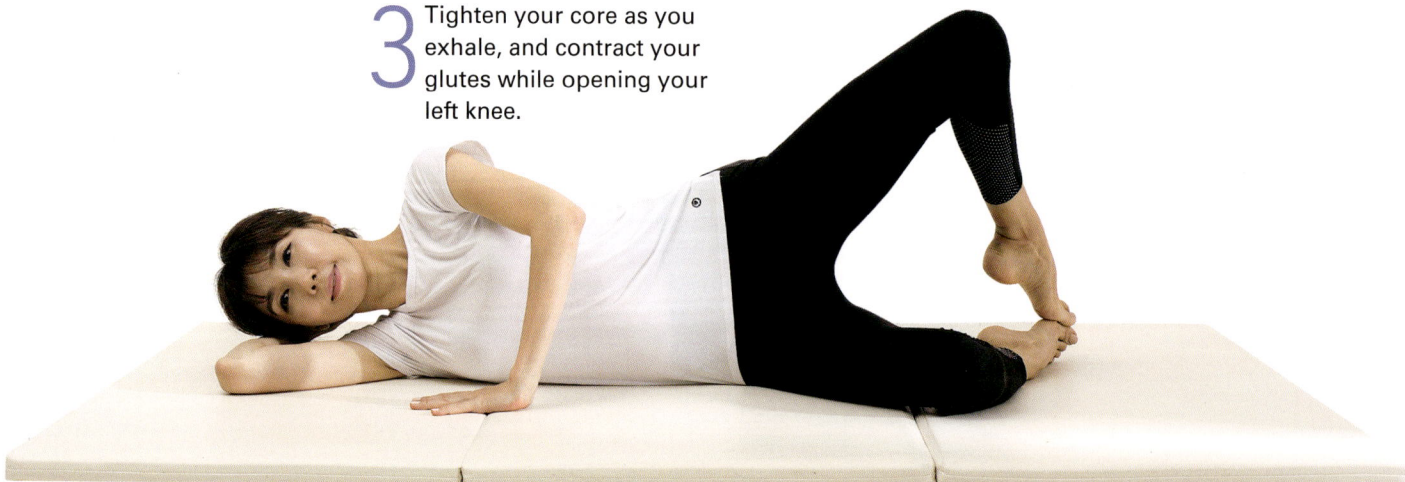

4 Return to the previous position as you inhale.

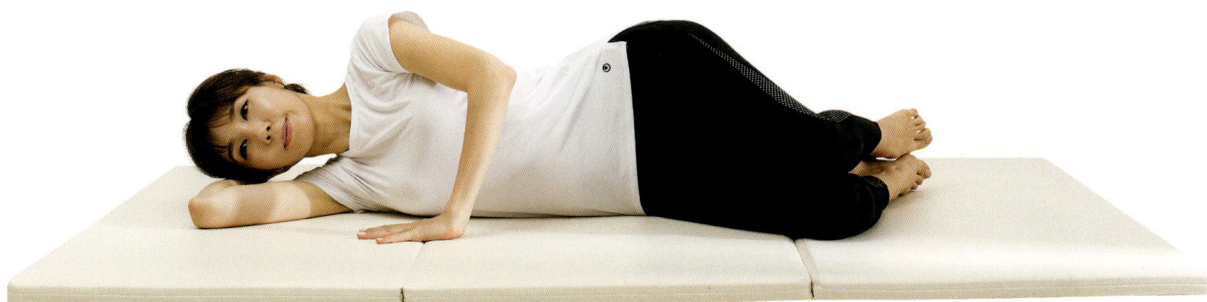

* Repeat movements 3 and 4 eight times on each side for three sets.

Maintain your spine alignment and focus on keeping your torso still.

Correct spine alignment with the core control. ✓

If you lose the core control, your neck might bend and your body might shake. X

Side-Lying Leg Lift

Side Lying 2

This exercise can strengthen the sides of your body, gently stretch the erector spinae muscle, strengthen the core, and tone your legs and hips.

1 Lie on your right side and place your left arm in front of your chest. Inhale to begin.

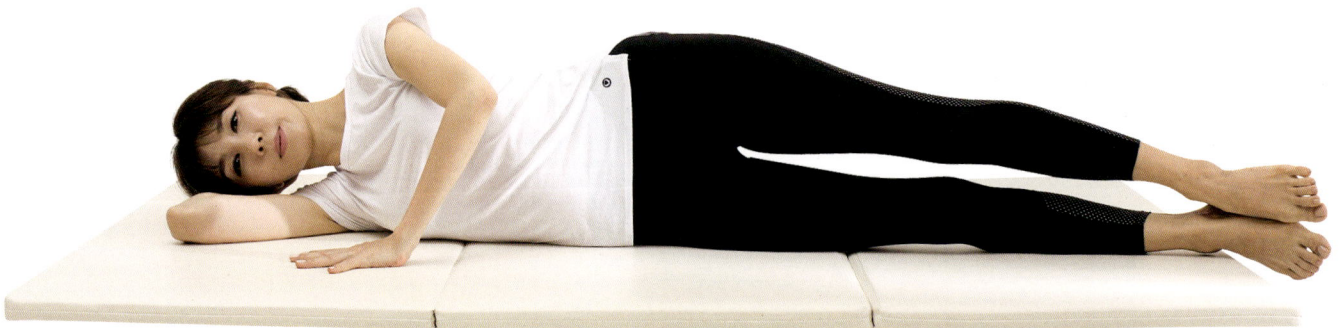

2 Raise your left leg as you exhale.

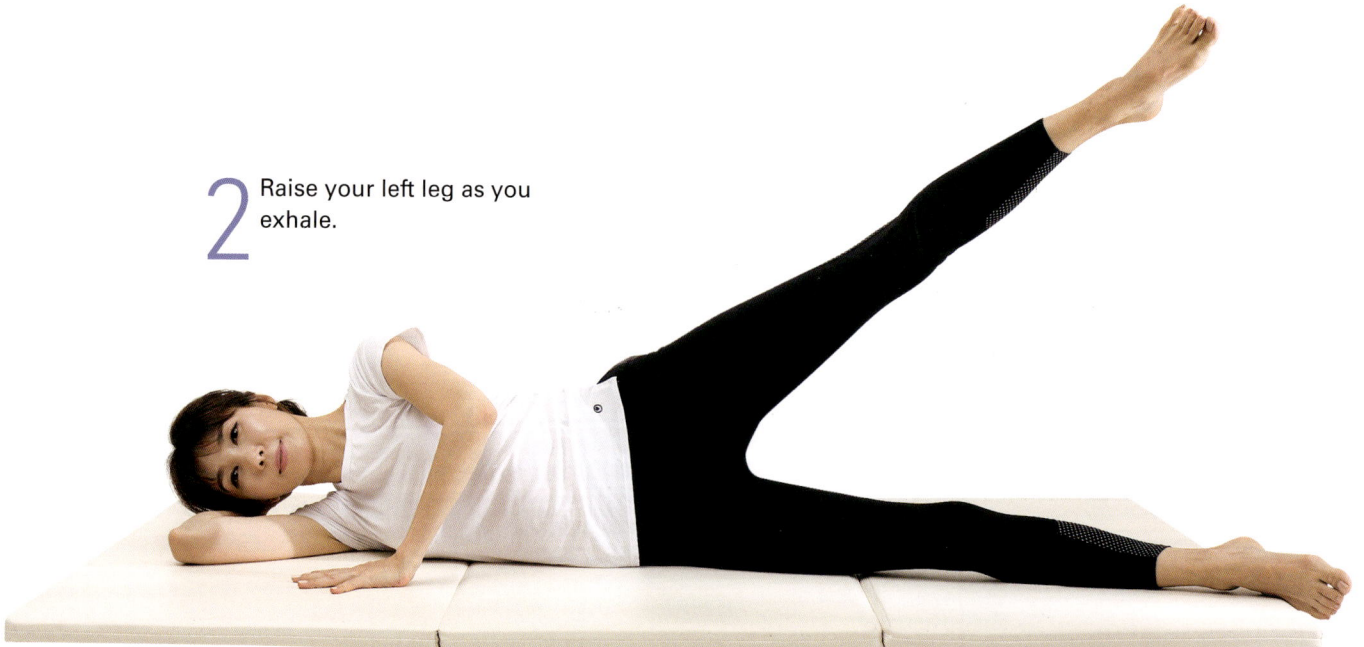

3 Lower your leg, bringing your legs together as you inhale.

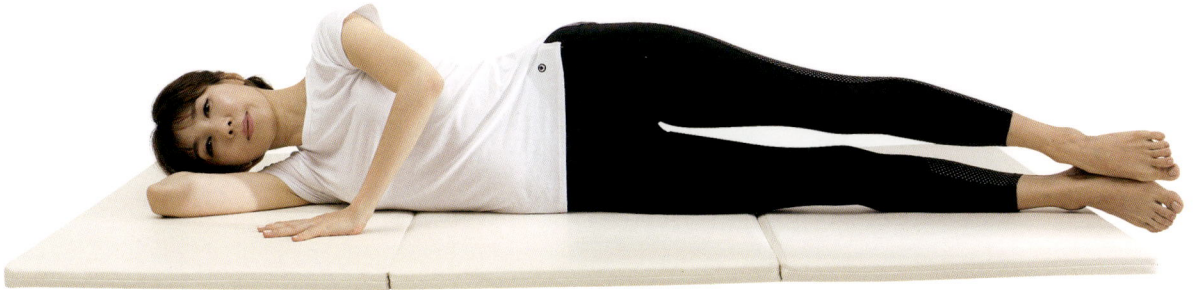

4 Lift up both legs as you exhale, and lower down as you inhale.

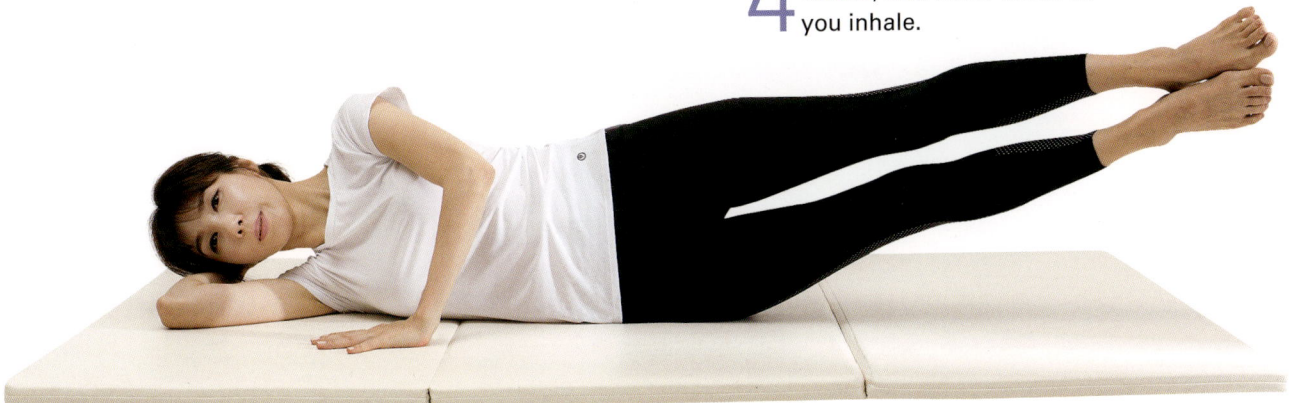

* Repeat movements 2 to 4 ten times on each side for two sets.

— Tip —

It's not important to raise your legs high. Focus on the movement of the lateral muscles throughout your body. Try not to overlift your legs, which can make you lose core control or bend your back. When you lift both legs, focus on keeping your balance.

Inner Thigh Lift

This exercise, which is beneficial to all body types, will sculpt and tone your legs. It also builds stability and control.

1 Lie on your right side with your hand supporting your head.

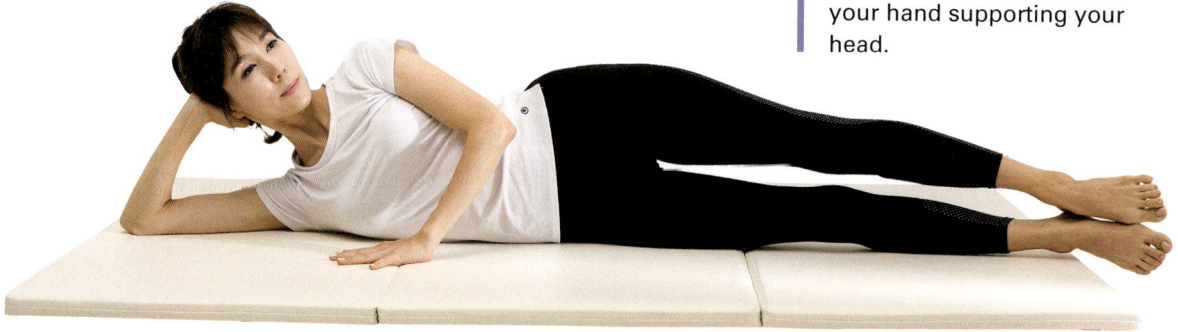

— Tip —

You can adjust your supporting arm according to your level.

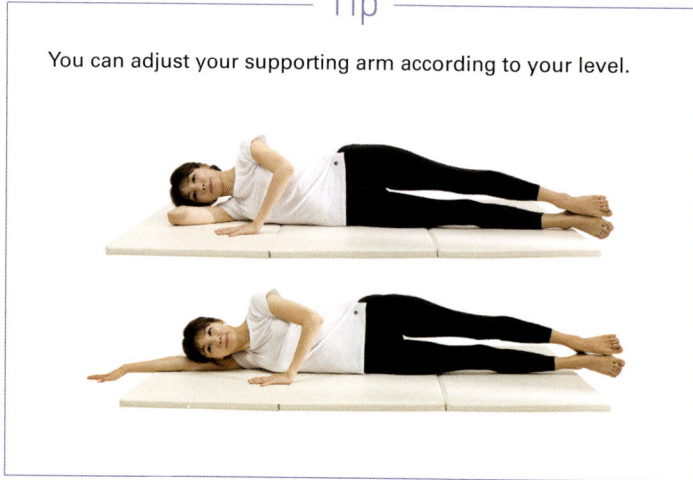

2 Bend and raise your left leg. Hold the ankle with your left arm.

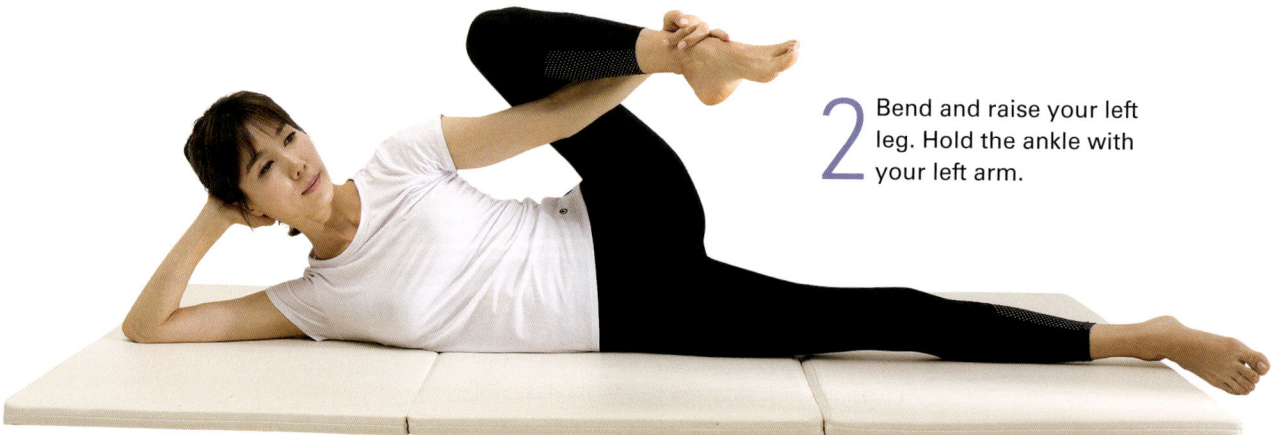

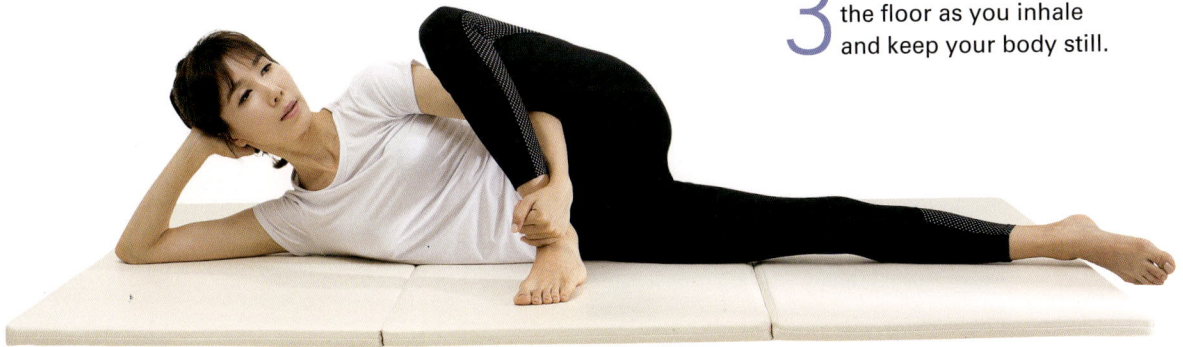

3 Place your left ankle on the floor as you inhale and keep your body still.

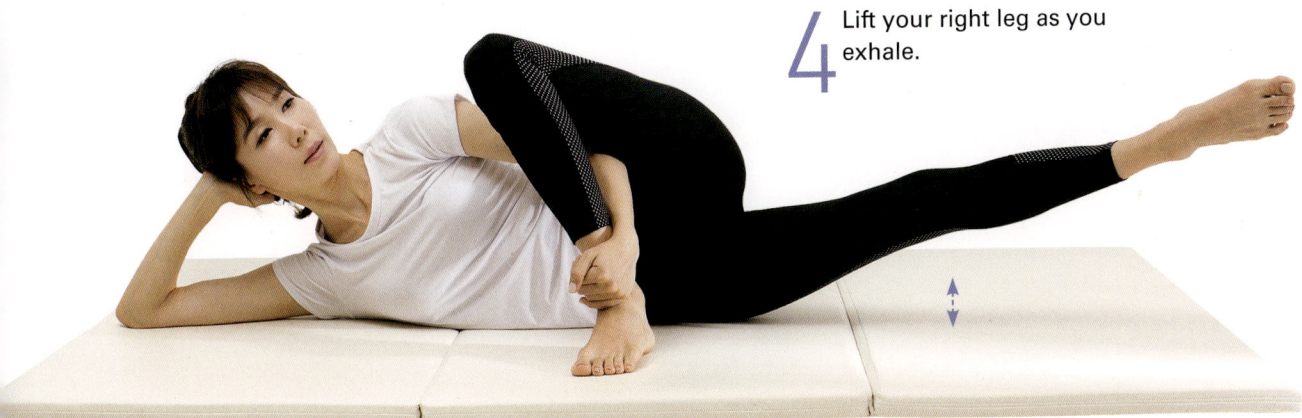

4 Lift your right leg as you exhale.

* Lift your leg up and down while exhaling in short breaths with each movement. Start on your right side for 10 repetitions, then on the left side for another 10. Repeat for three sets.

── Tip ──

Lift your leg up and down with light, continuous movements, focusing on keeping your torso stable and still.

Side-Lying Kick

The motion of bringing your legs back and forth improves lower-body balance and flexibility. It also tones your hips.

1 Stabilize your body on the floor by supporting your head with your right arm and pressing into the floor with your left hand for balance.

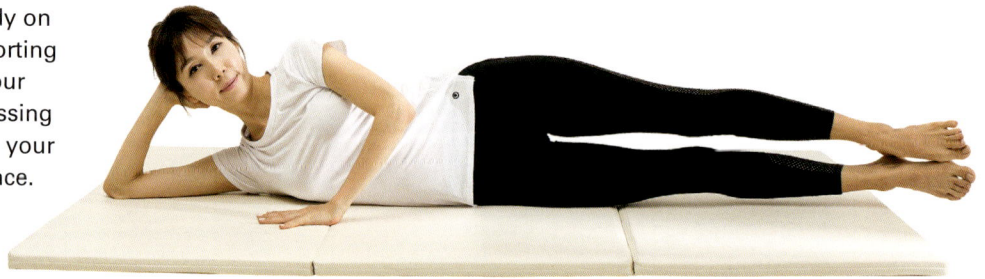

2 Kick your left leg forward as you inhale, flexing the foot.

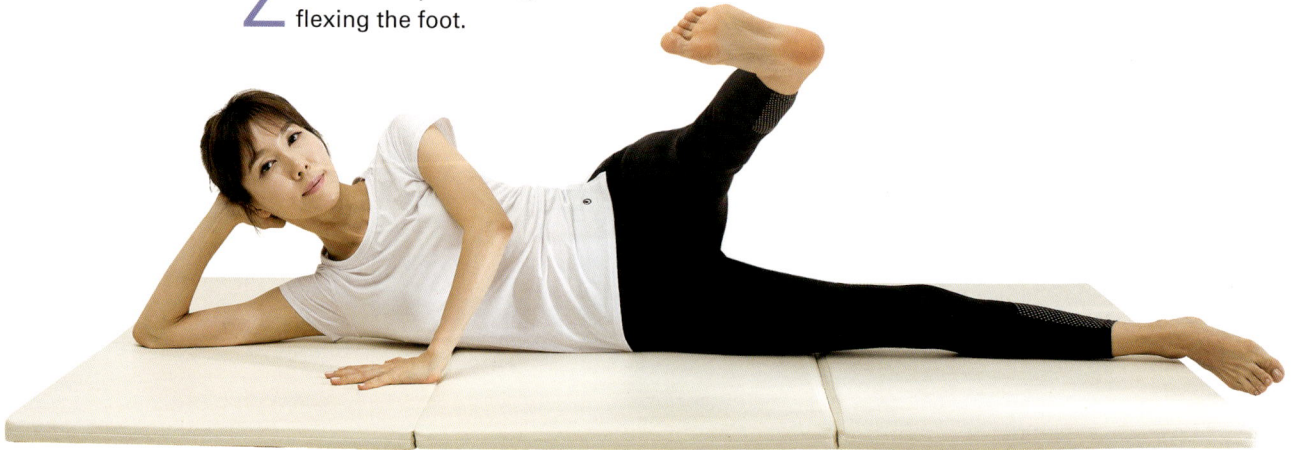

3 Kick your left leg behind you as you exhale, and stretch the ankle.

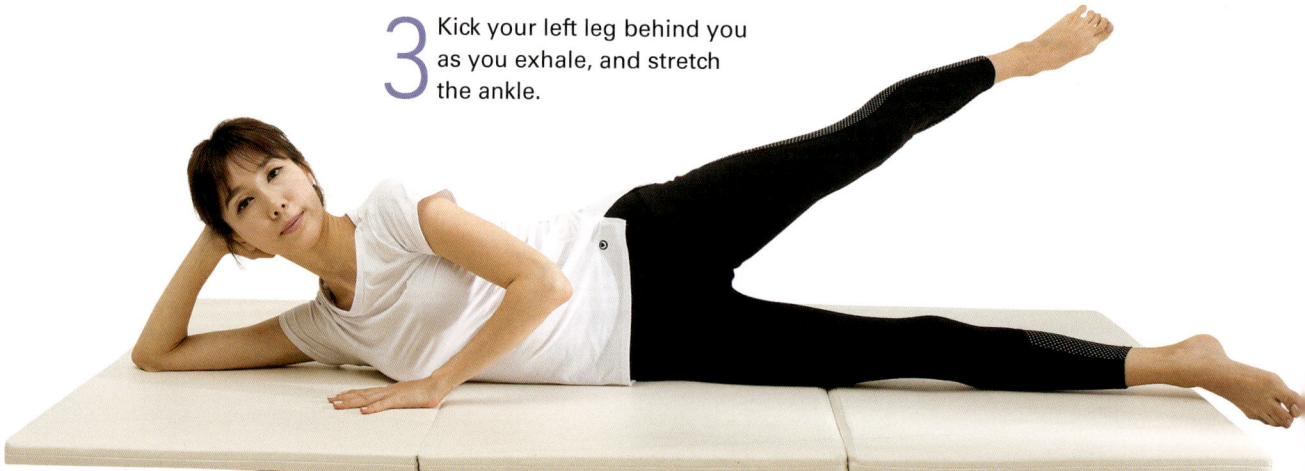

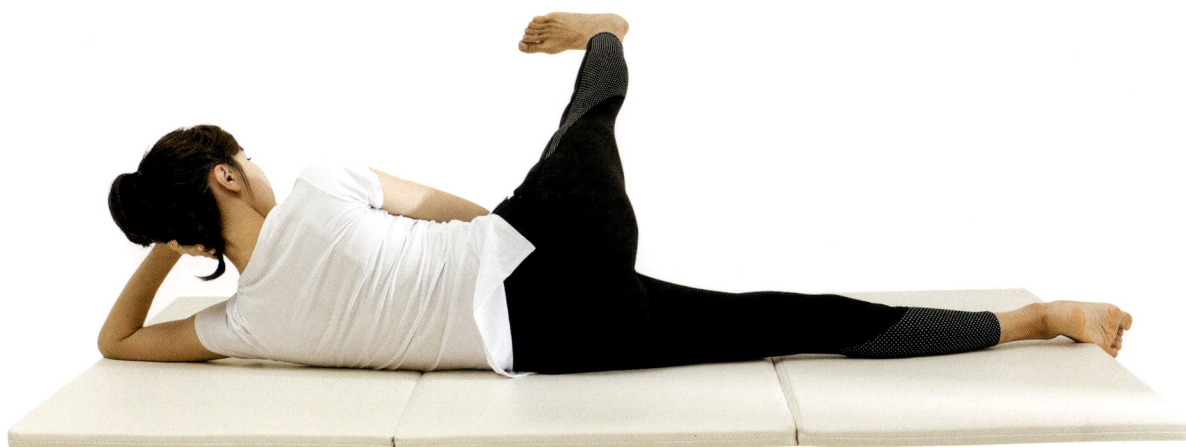

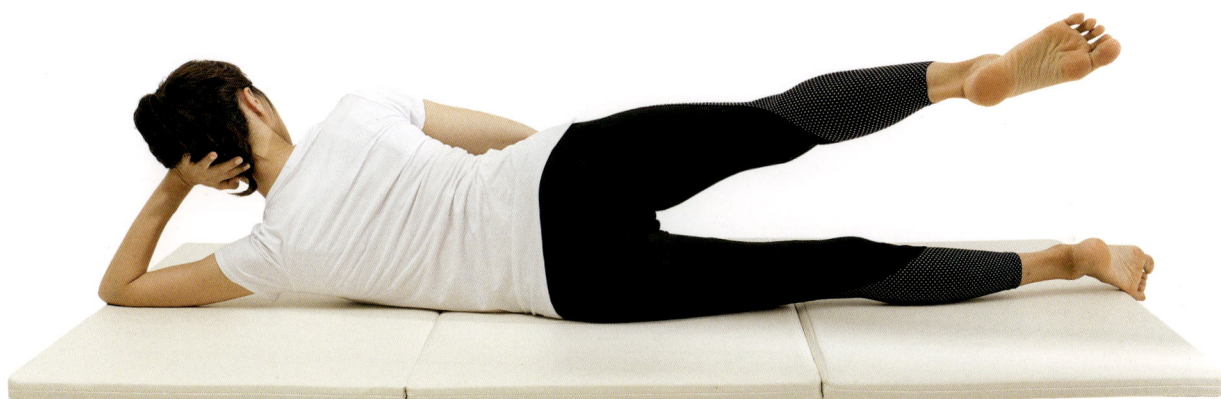

* Kick your leg back and forth eight times, then alternate legs.

─── Tip ───

Control your core as you breathe to avoid using the momentum you get when you swing your legs. Breathing should help you move as you inhale and exhale.

Side Lying 5

Long Leg Lift

This exercise improves flexibility and core balance. It also supports lower-body circulation and helps reduce weight.

1 Lie on your right side with your hand supporting your head. Inhale to begin.

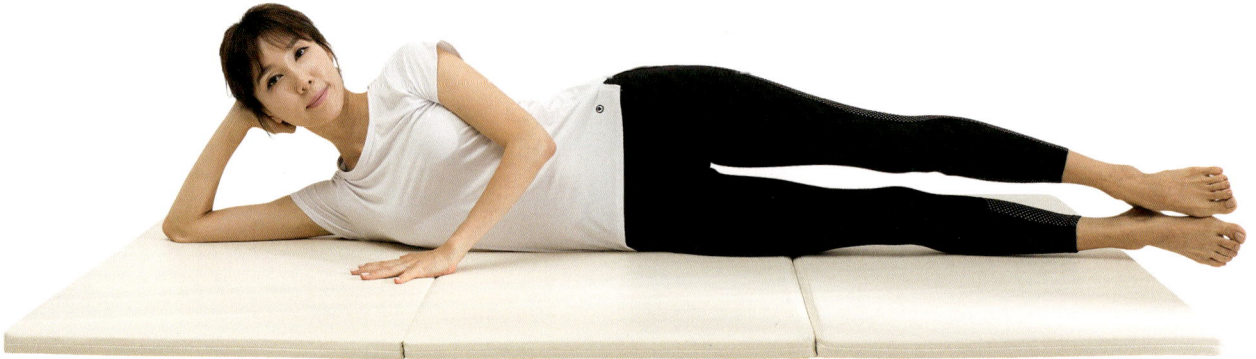

2 Raise your left leg high to the side as you exhale.

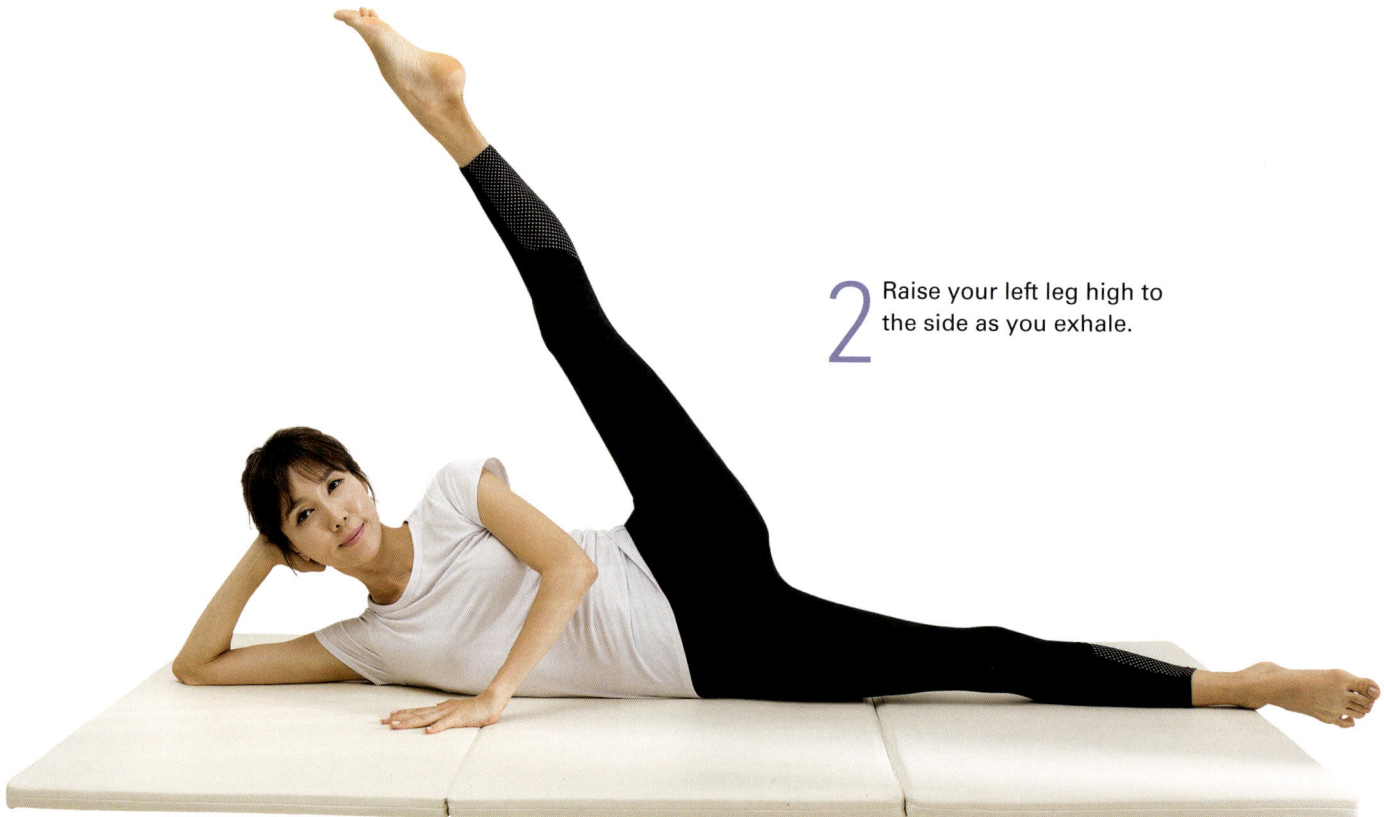

58

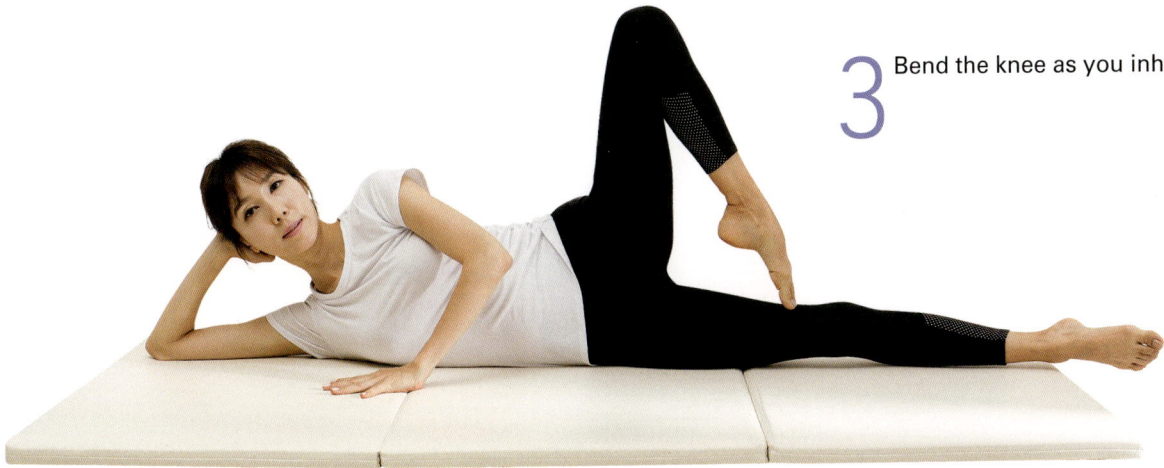

3 Bend the knee as you inhale.

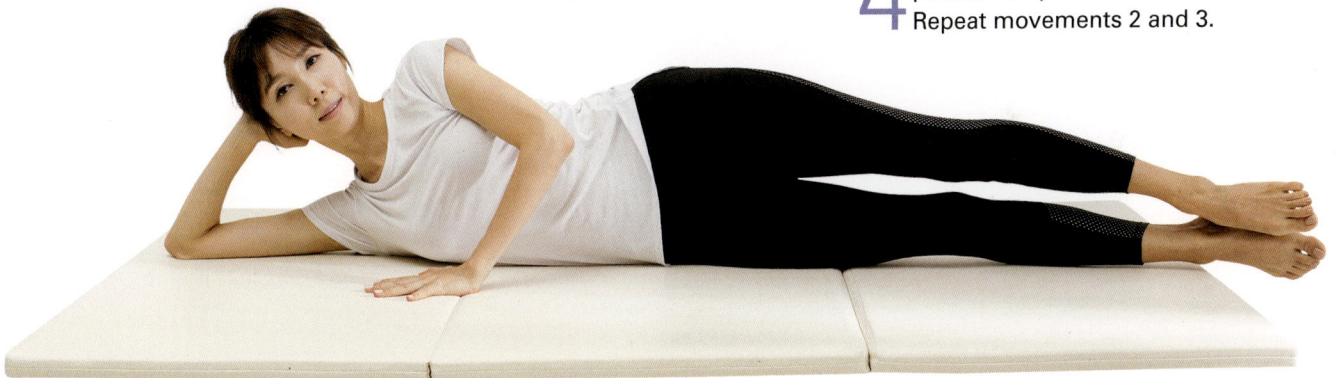

4 Return to the starting position as you exhale. Repeat movements 2 and 3.

* Repeat three sets of movements 2 and 3 on alternate legs.

--- Tip ---

The key to this movement is using the strength of the lifting leg. If you focus only on kicking your leg up, you might bend your knee or strain the ligament. Focus on the back of your leg to lengthen and control the motion as you lift.

Prone

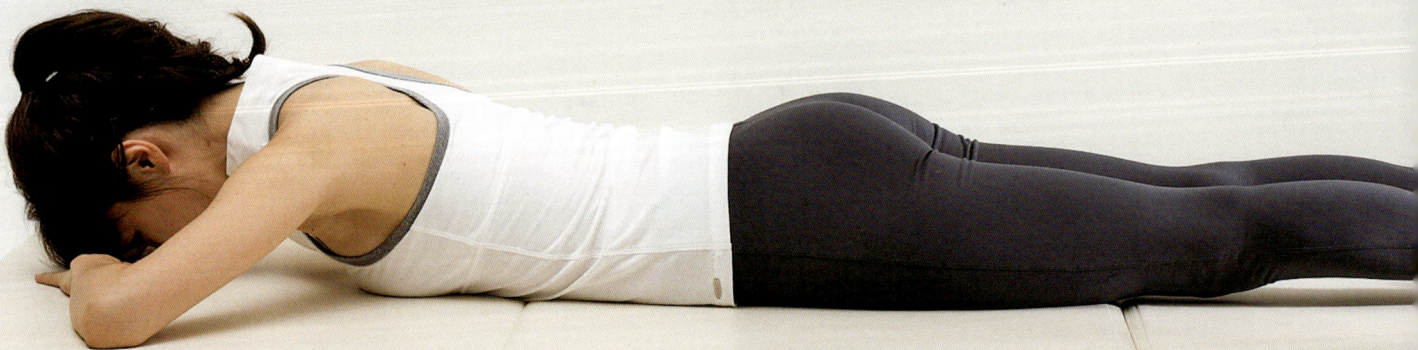

Neutral Posture

Most exercises in the prone position require you to engage your spine or lift up your torso and lower body. Avoid overtightening or overarching your back beyond your ability. It's important to maintain the natural curve of the spine and engage your abdomen and back with the proper tension. Also, make sure to keep your stomach lifted and activate your core.

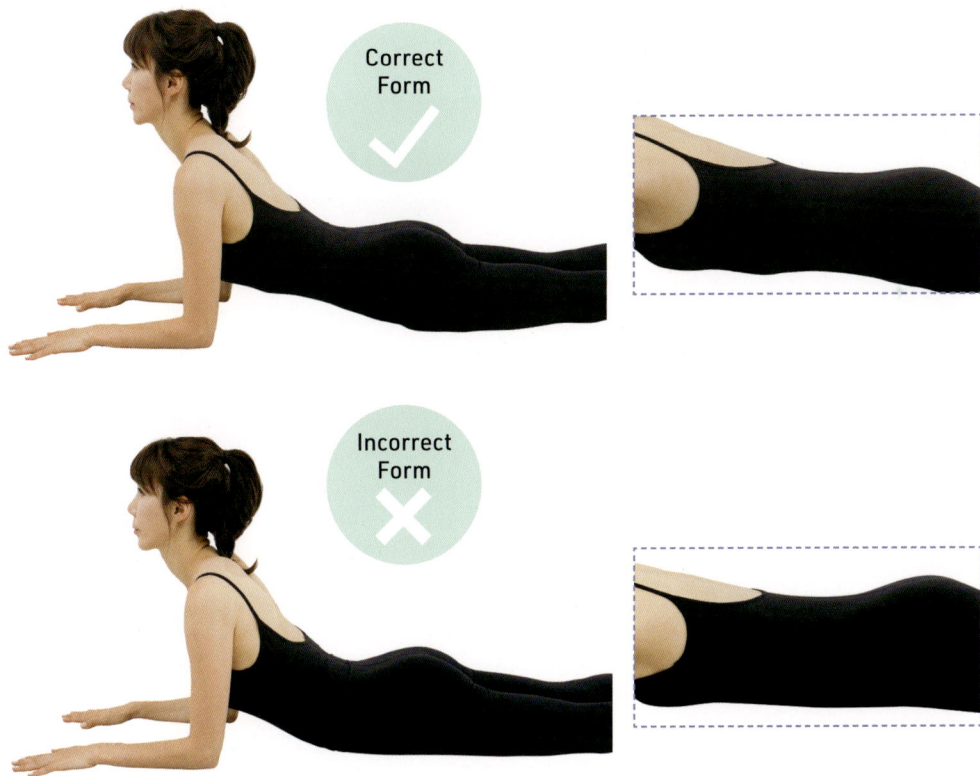

Correct
Form
✓

Incorrect
Form
✗

The Sphinx

This exercise can correct neck and spine alignment without straining the back.

1 Start in the prone position with your legs pelvis-width apart and place your forehead on your hands, touching the floor.

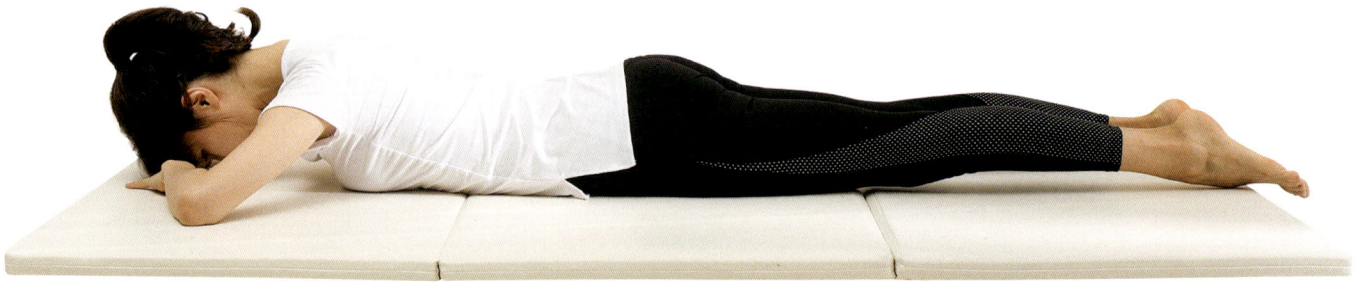

2 Lift your torso slowly, starting from your head. Place your elbows under your shoulders with your forearms on the mat to make the sphinx position.

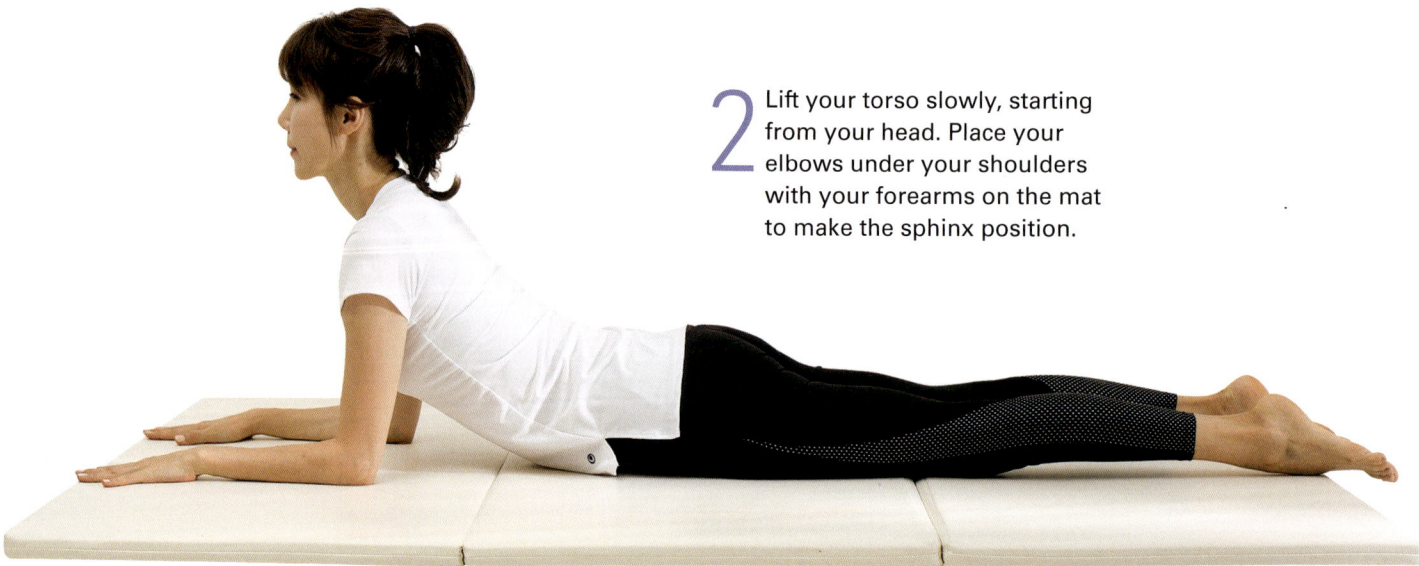

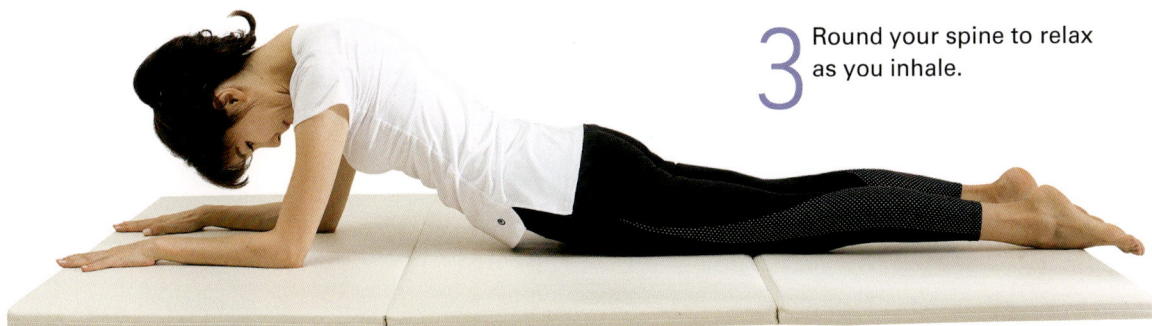

3 Round your spine to relax as you inhale.

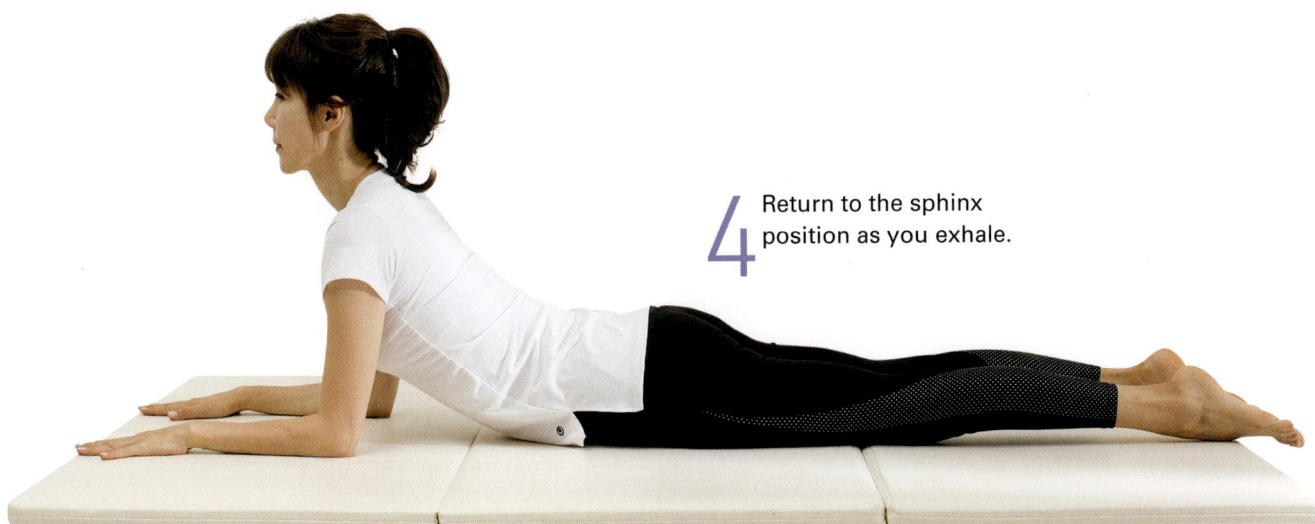

4 Return to the sphinx position as you exhale.

* Repeat movements 3 and 4 eight times to round the spine and lift the torso. Complete two sets.

Tip

This movement can engage your spine in a way similar to cat pose. It doesn't require dynamic motion, but gets excellent results. Focus on contracting and releasing your muscles according to your ability, and do not overstrain your spine.

Leg Raise

This exercise can strengthen the erector spinae and core muscles. It can also tone your hips and support leg alignment.

1 Lie on your belly with your feet touching each other. Place your forehead on your hands, touching the floor. Inhale to begin.

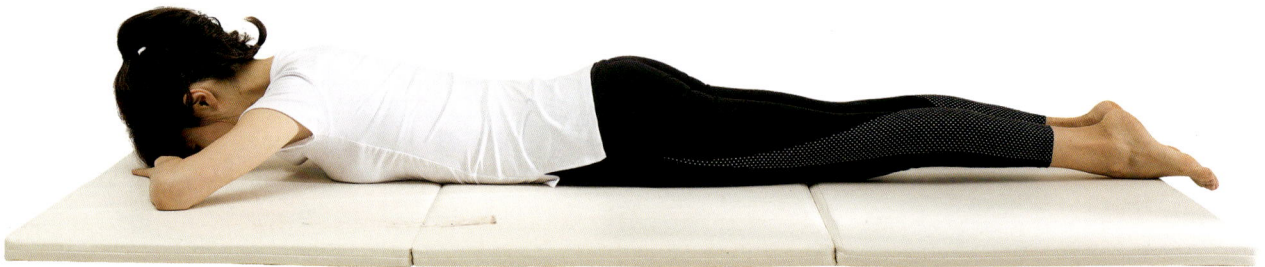

2 Lift up both legs while tightening your abdomen as you exhale.

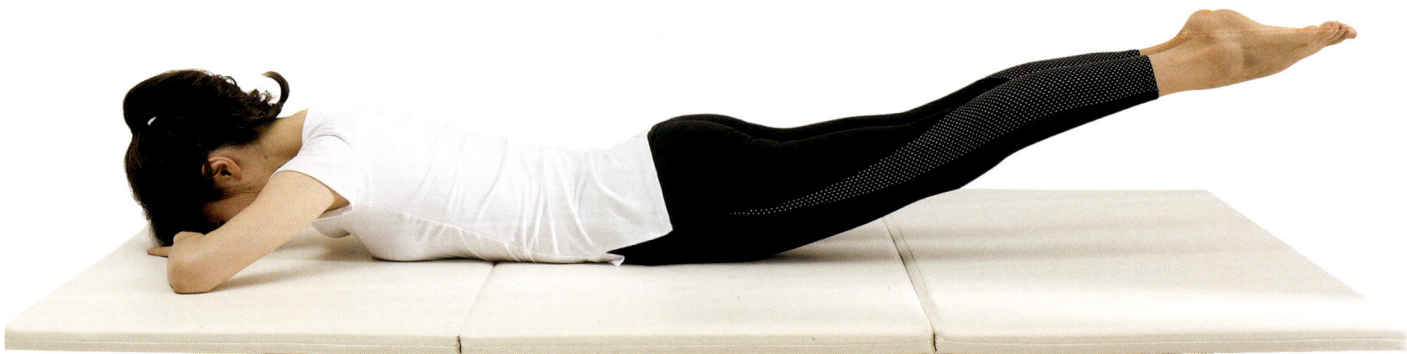

3 Lower your legs without touching the floor as you inhale.

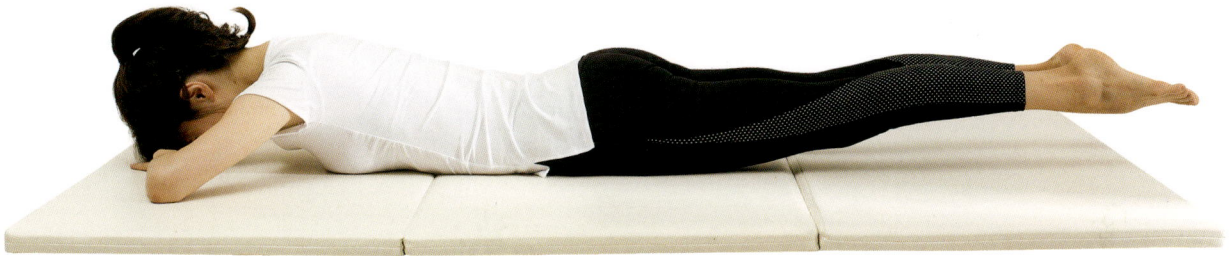

4 Lift up your legs as you exhale, and lower your legs as you inhale. Keep the tension in your abdomen. Repeat several times.

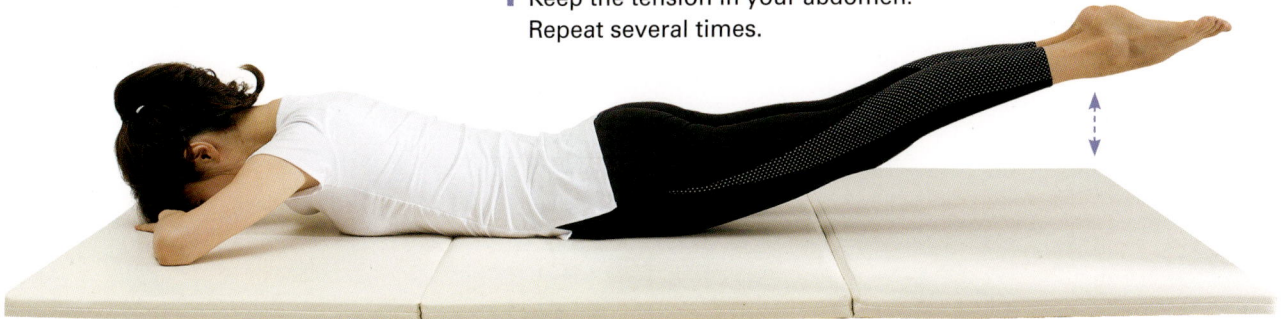

* Repeat lifting your legs up and down eight times for two sets.

Tip

When exercising in a prone position, focus on keeping your abdominal muscles engaged at all times. The goal is to reach out with your legs away from your body, not to lift them high.

Swimming

This exercise engages muscles throughout the entire body, with a focus on core strength and the erector spinae muscles. It helps build strong glutes and supports spinal alignment.

1 Lie on your belly and reach both arms forward as you inhale.

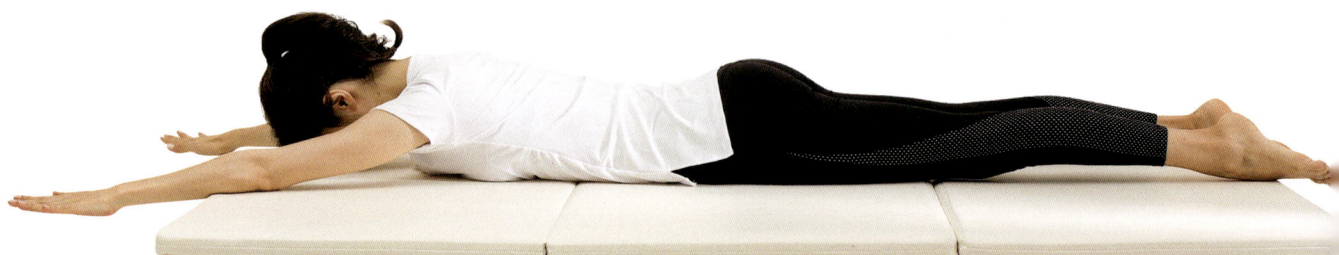

2 Lift up the right arm and the left leg as you exhale.

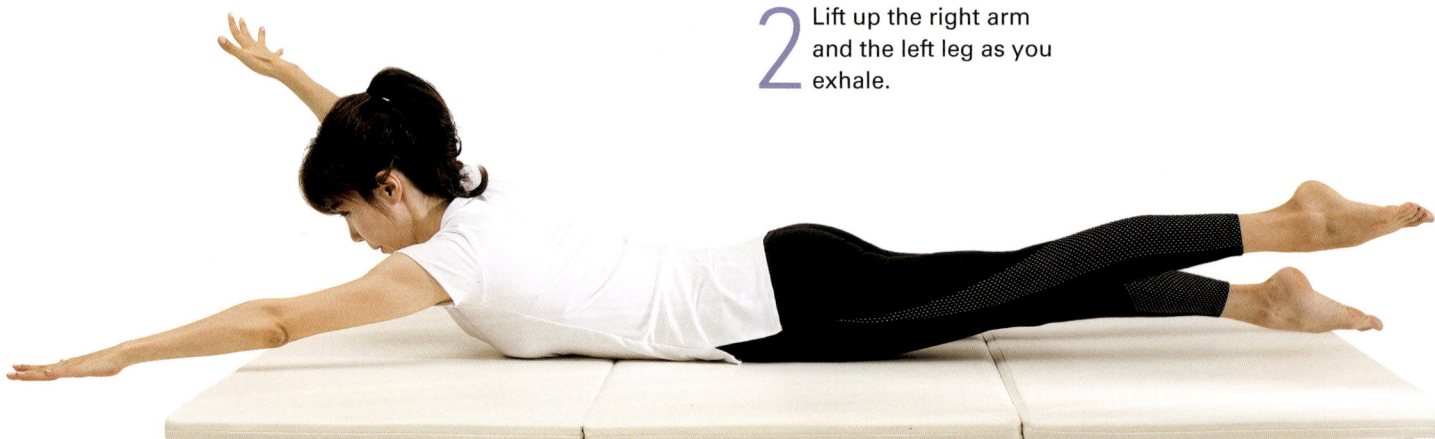

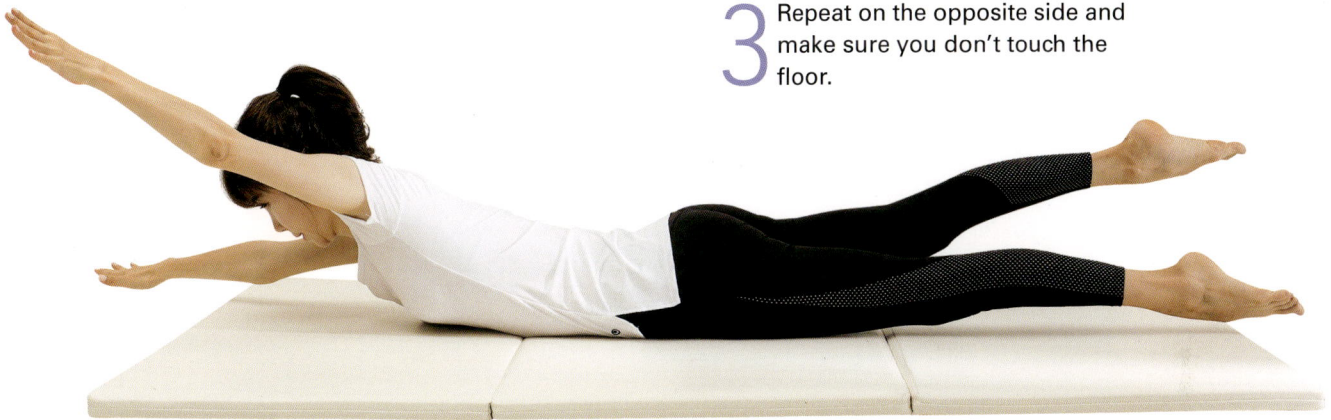

3 Repeat on the opposite side and make sure you don't touch the floor.

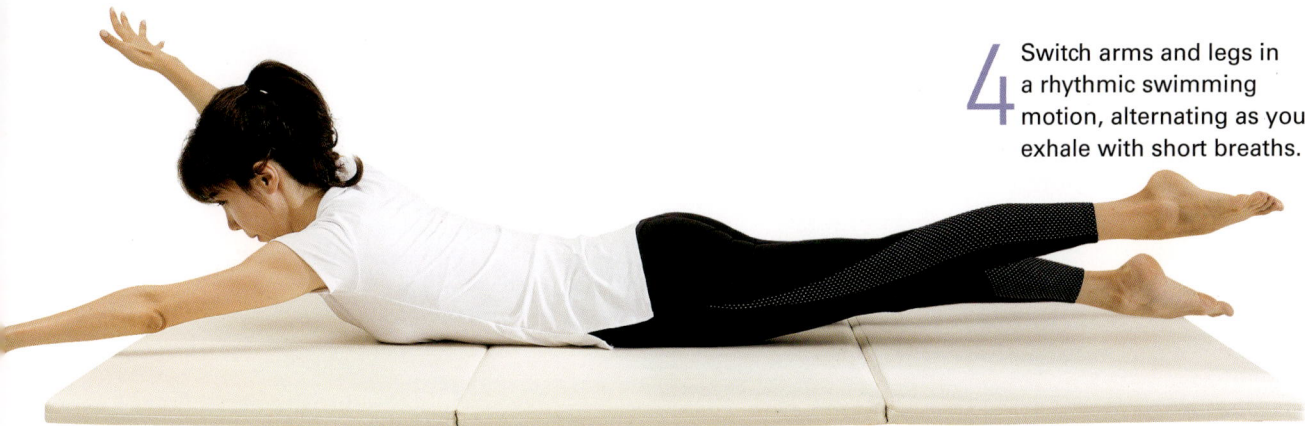

4 Switch arms and legs in a rhythmic swimming motion, alternating as you exhale with short breaths.

* Repeat the movement eight times on each side for three sets.

Tip

Pay attention to your body's movements and maintain the tension from head to toe. If you release the tension, your gaze may lift, your shoulders may tense, and your body may shake. Focus on your breathing and be aware of your spine.

The Swan

This exercise can strengthen the posterior regions of shoulders, back, and hips. It can also tone the back and trim the waistline.

1 Lie flat on your belly with both arms bent at your sides and the legs pelvis-width apart.

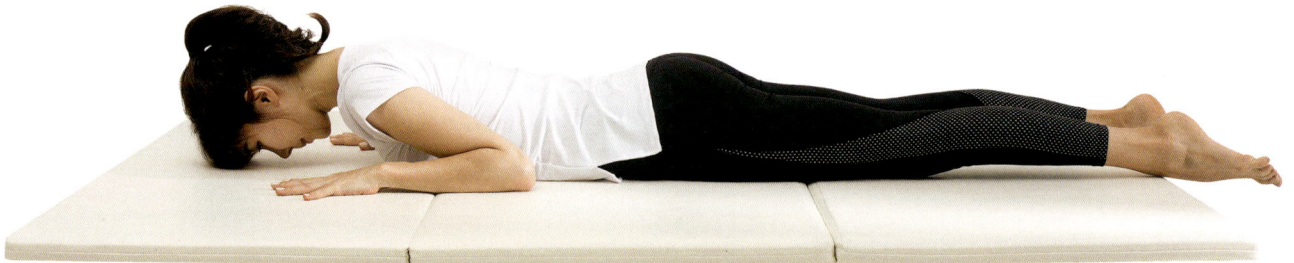

2 Raise your torso as much as you can while inhaling.

* Your pelvis should stay slightly off the floor, but if you lack flexibility or have pain in your back, only raise to where you feel comfortable.

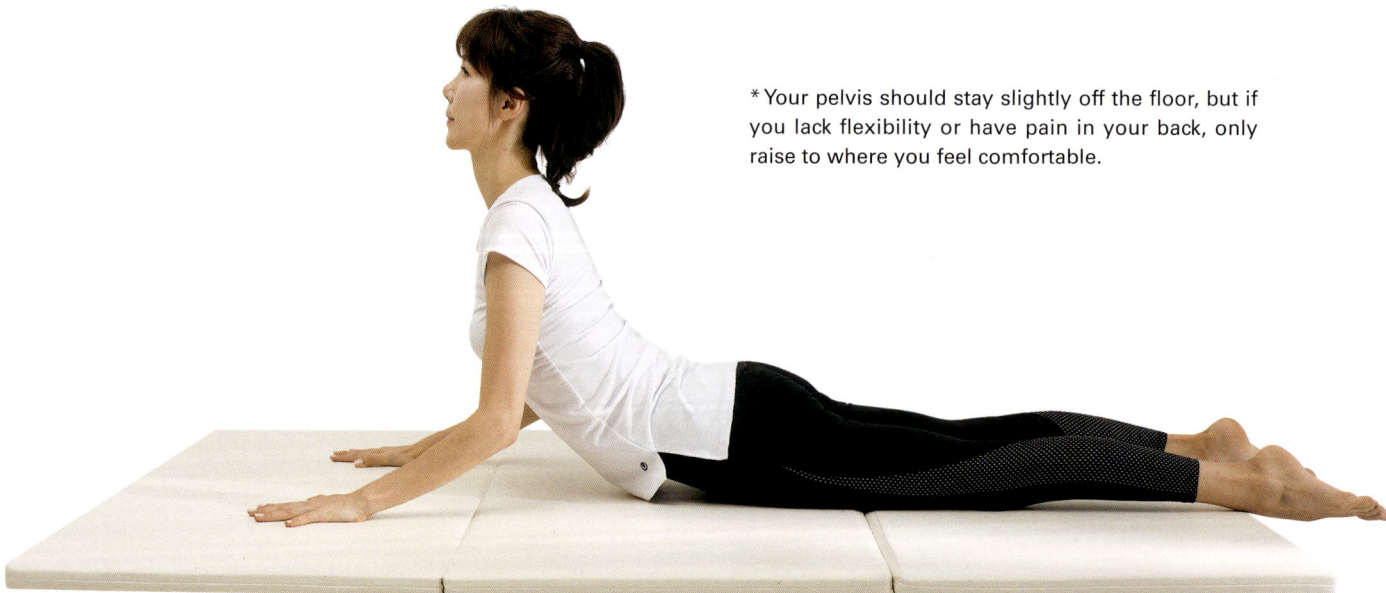

3 Tighten your core and hips as you reach your arms forward and raise your legs as you exhale.

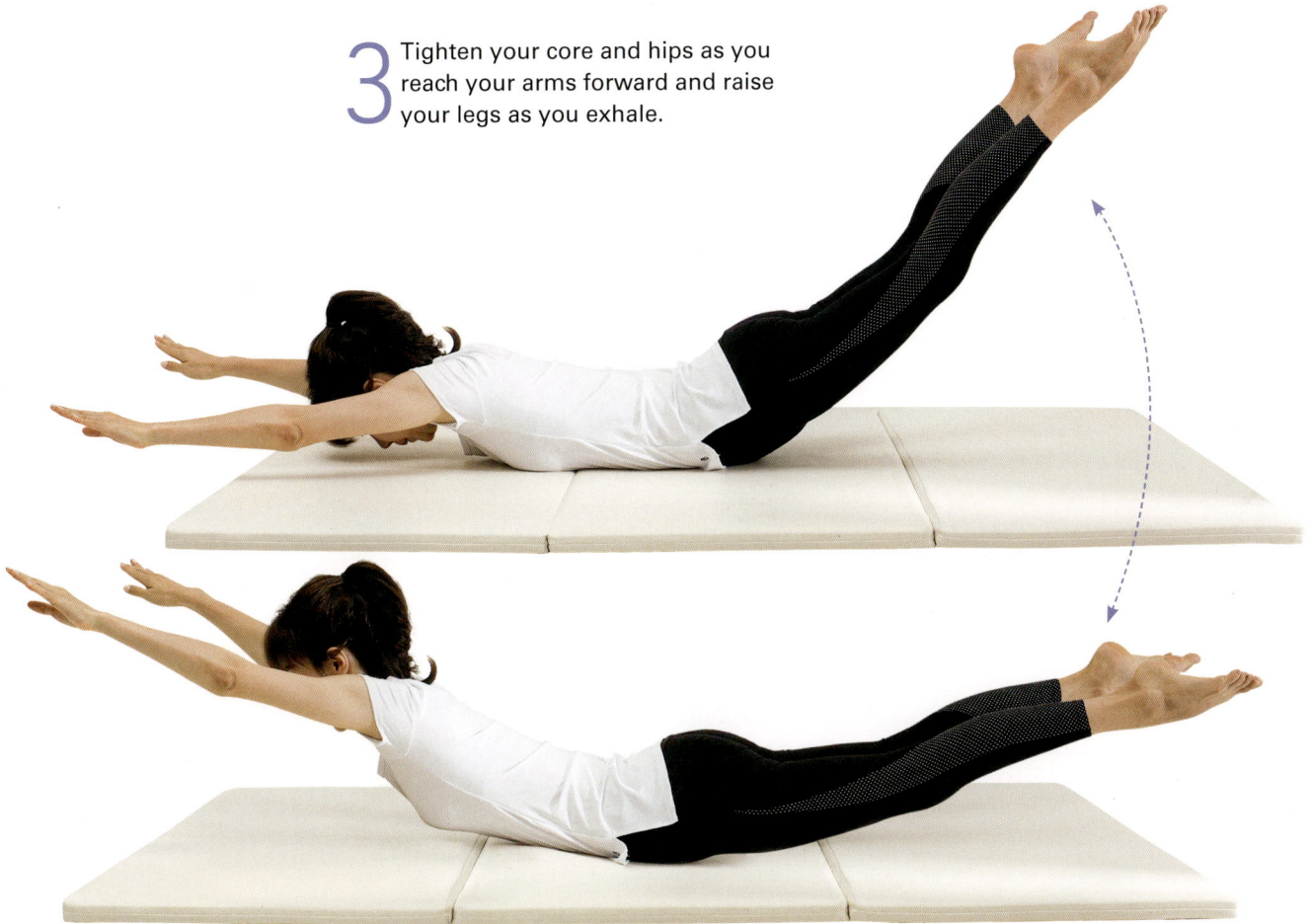

4 Rock back and forth like a roly-poly toy as you inhale and exhale.

* Repeat the movement six times for two sets.

Tip

If you raise your arms and legs too high, it may cause your head to drop, placing strain on your back. Stay focused to avoid overextending, and pay attention to your core.

Double Kick

This exercise can strengthen the posterior regions of the body by correcting the spine, and it can tone the hips and thighs.

1 Lie flat on your belly with your legs touching each other. Place your forehead on your hands, touching the floor. Inhale to begin.

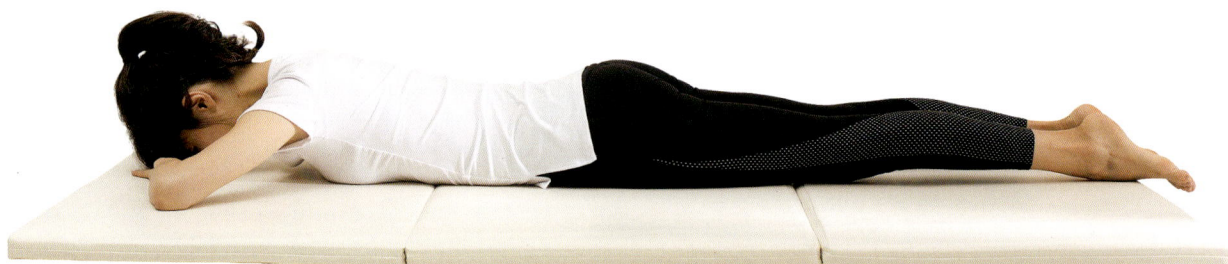

2 Bend your knees twice, taking a short breath with each bend. Point your toes during the first bend, then flex your feet on the second.

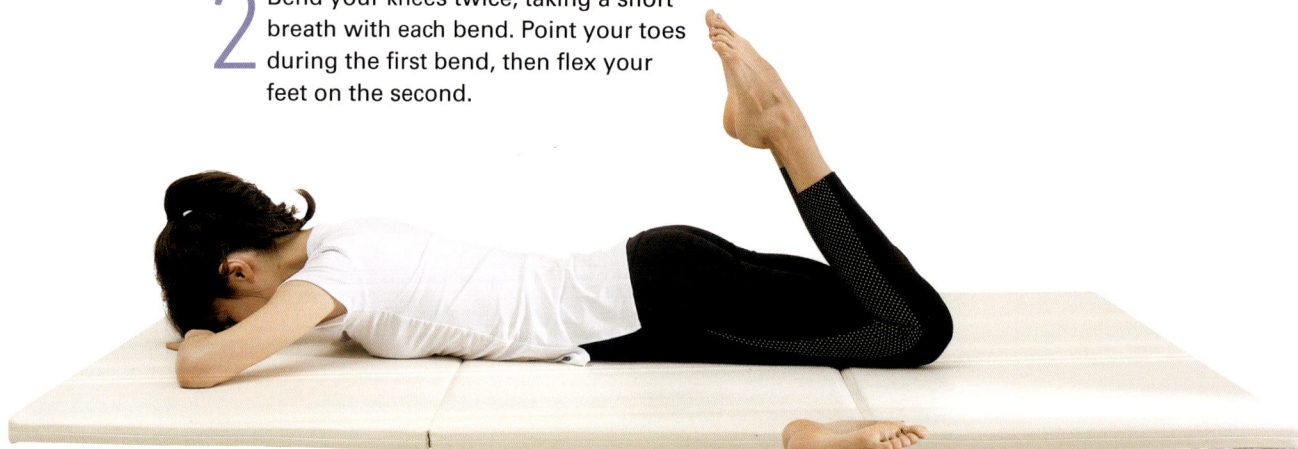

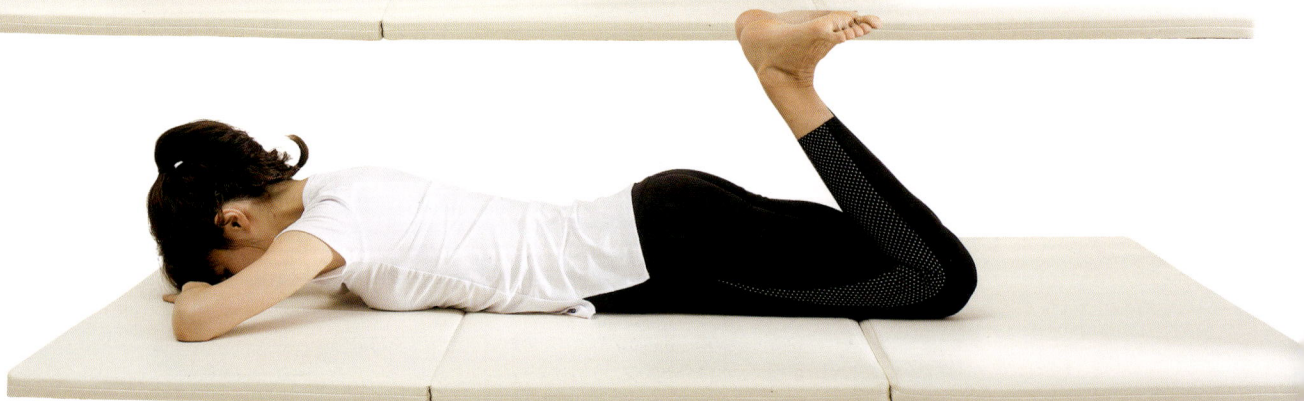

3 Extend both legs, keeping them tight as you inhale again.

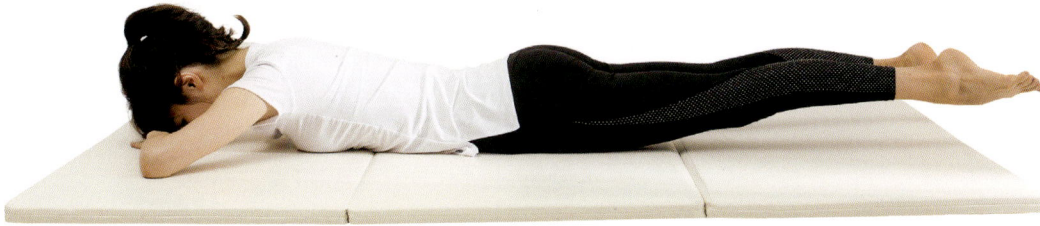

4 Tighten the core and the hips as you exhale and spread your legs.

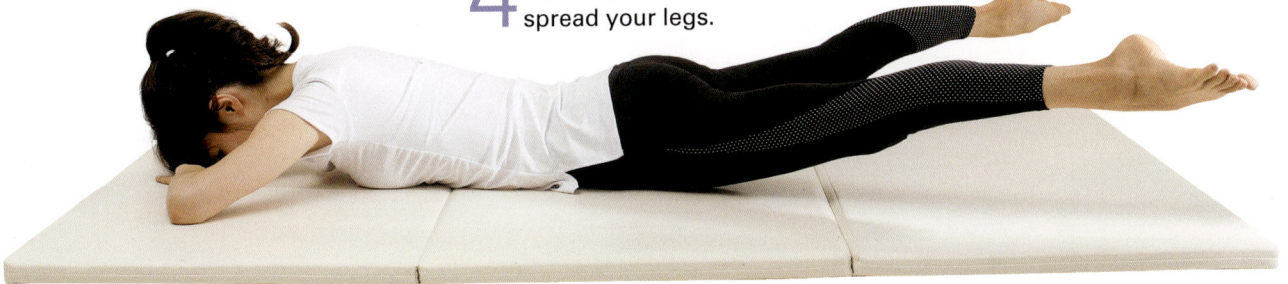

5 Return to the starting position as you inhale.

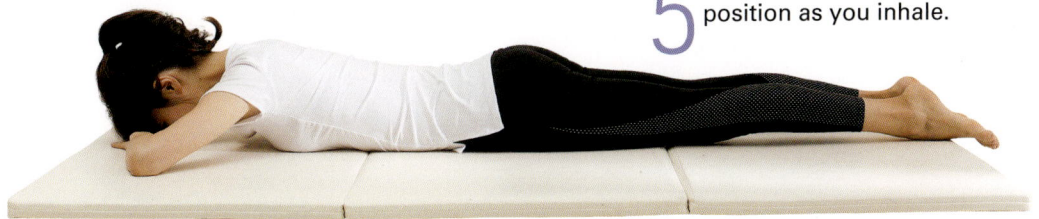

* Repeat six sets of movements 2 to 5, bending the knees and ankles then extending and spreading the legs.

— Tip —

Remember the correct order of the movement to better understand how your muscles work and to smoothly connect each step with body awareness.

AllFours

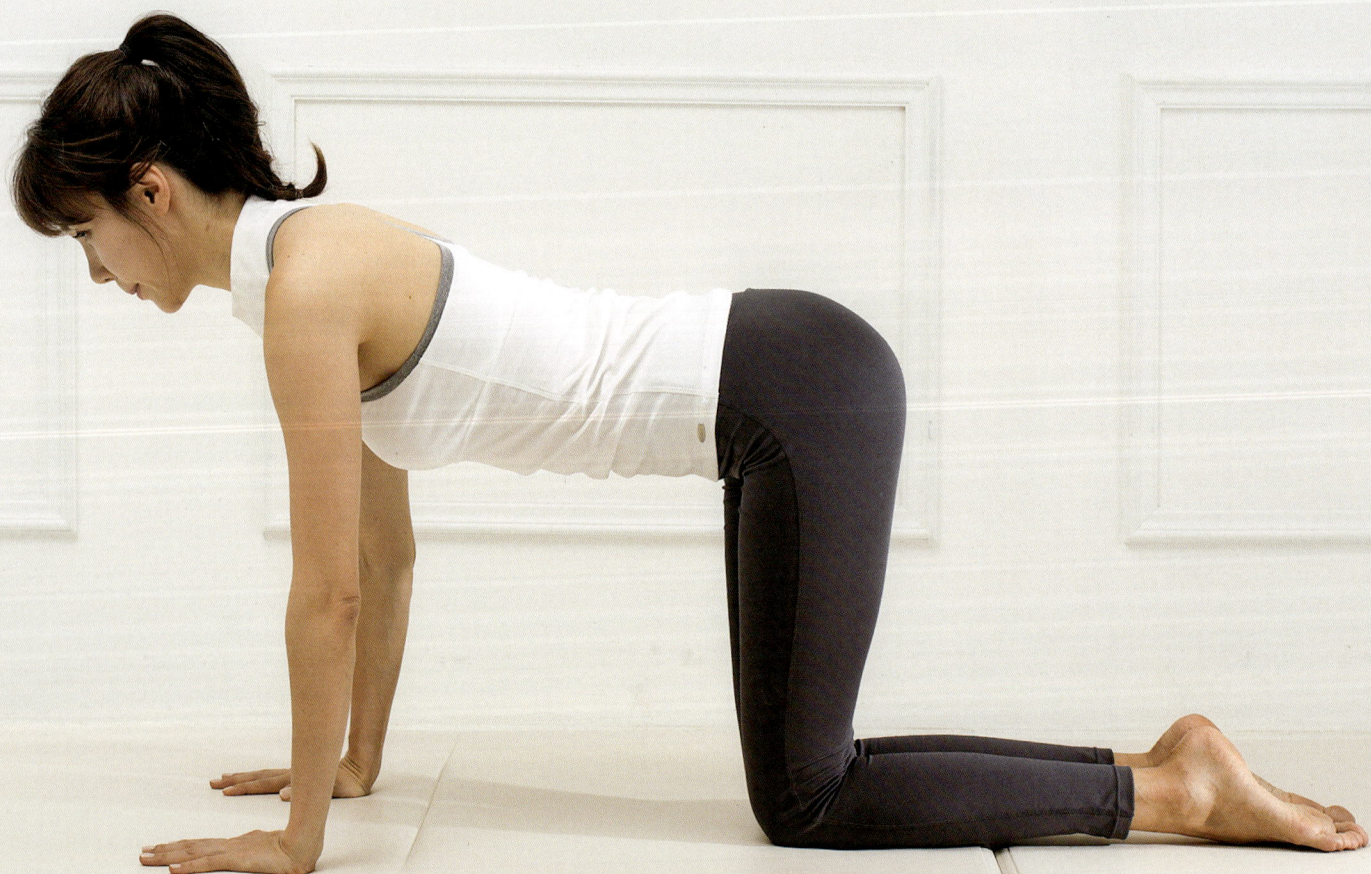

Neutral Posture

The all-fours position counteracts many problems caused by upright walking by aligning the spine and strengthening the muscles around it, improving flexibility and strength. Be mindful of your wrists and elbows—evenly distribute your weight over your palms. Try not to overstrain your abdomen.

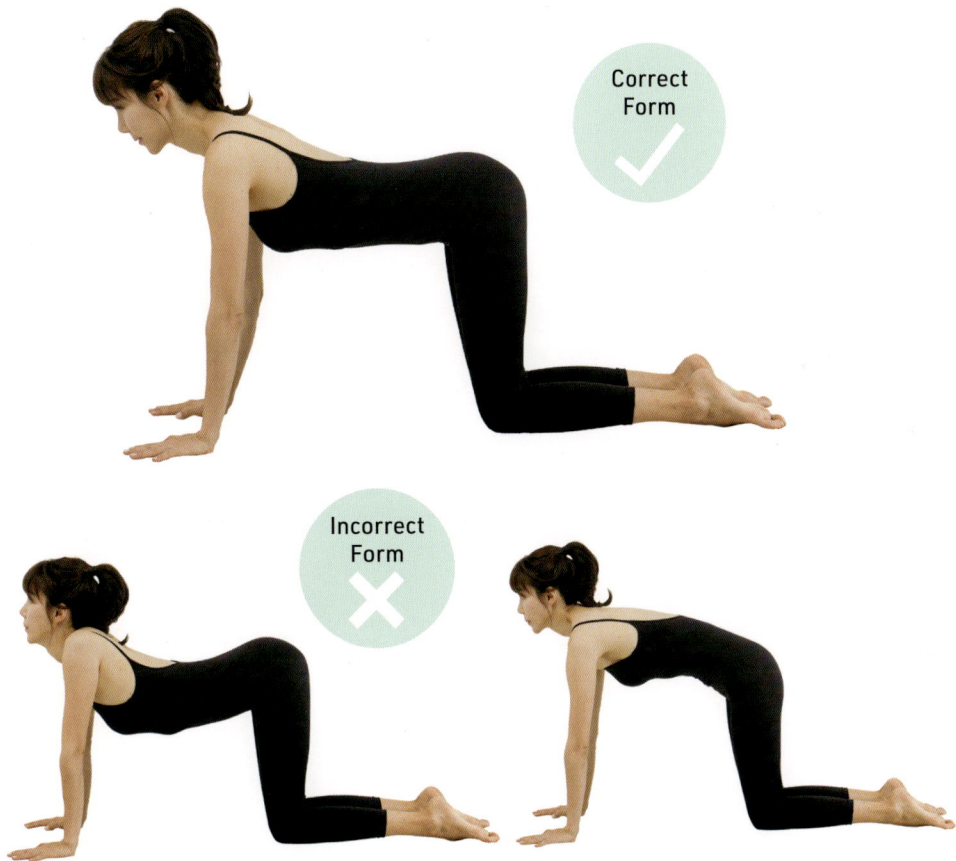

Correct Form ✓

Incorrect Form ✗

Cat Stretch

This exercise may help with scoliosis correction. Practicing this stretch with mindful Pilates breathing promotes a smooth, supple spine.

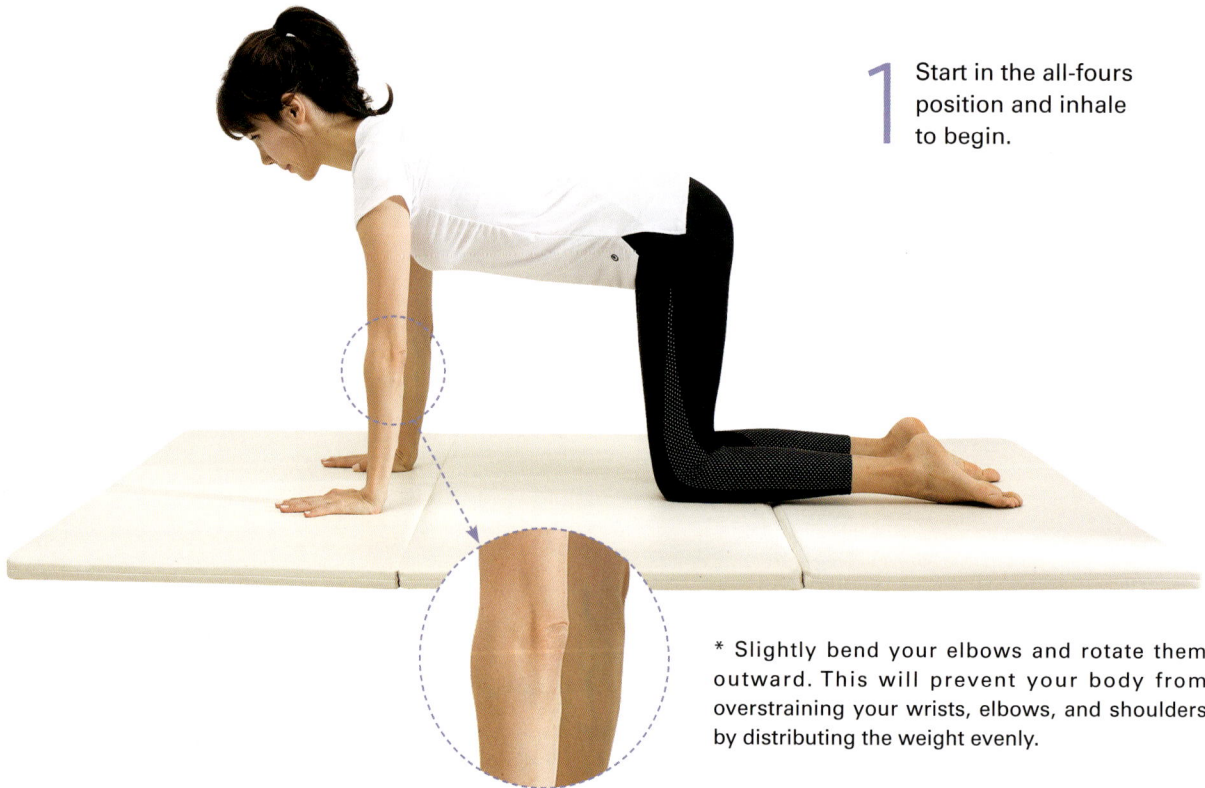

1 Start in the all-fours position and inhale to begin.

* Slightly bend your elbows and rotate them outward. This will prevent your body from overstraining your wrists, elbows, and shoulders by distributing the weight evenly.

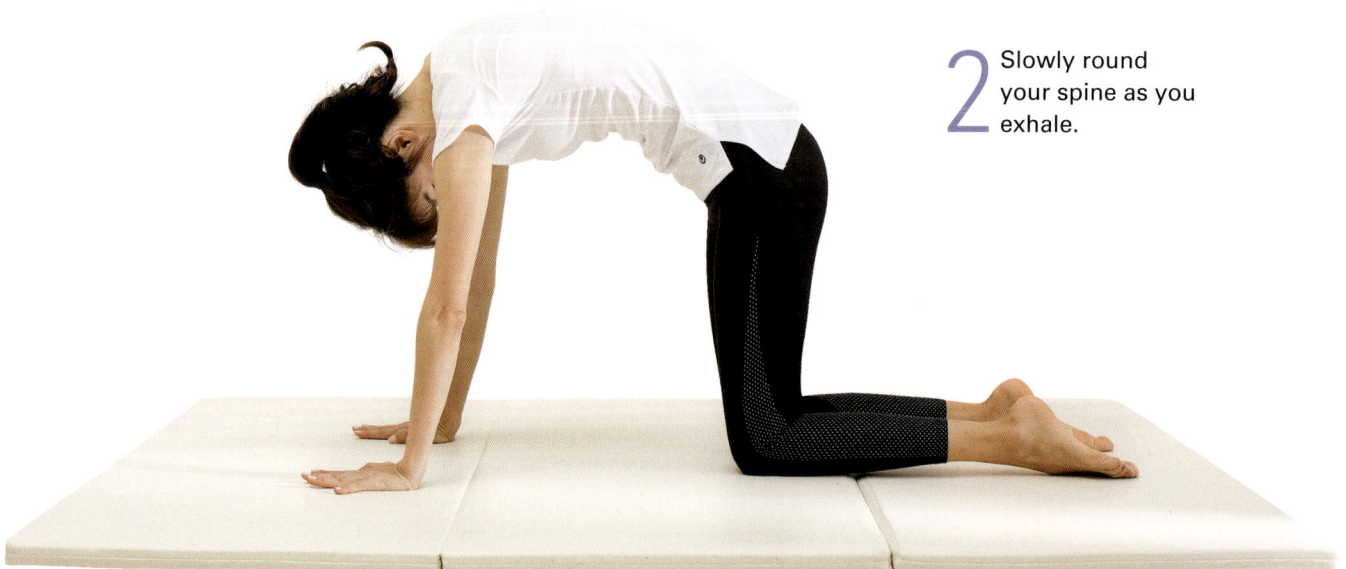

2 Slowly round your spine as you exhale.

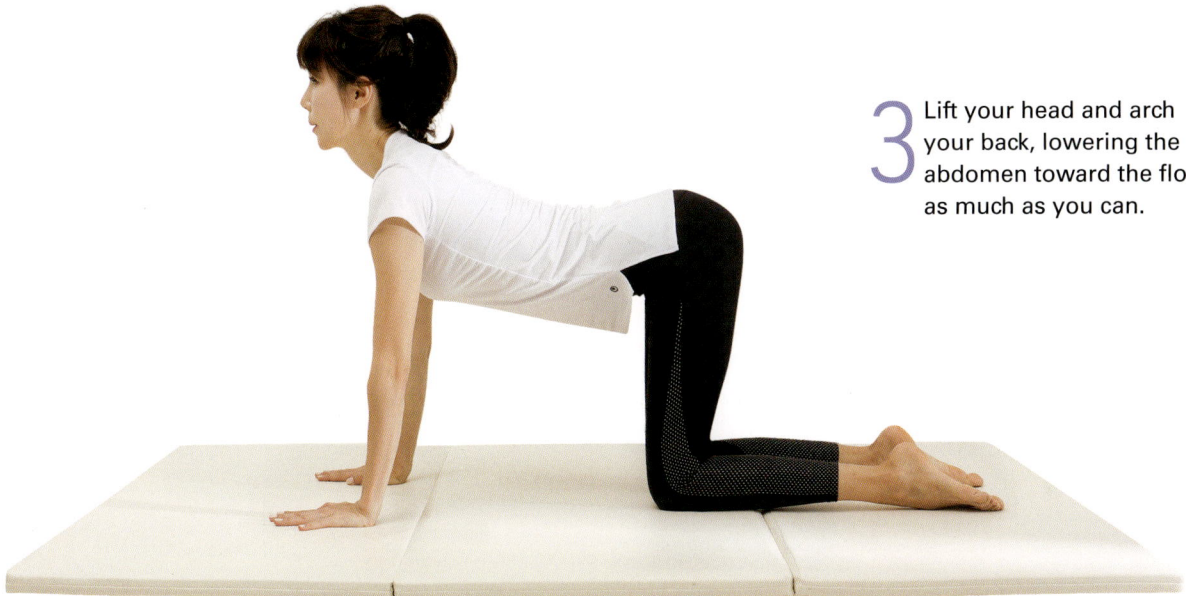

3 Lift your head and arch your back, lowering the abdomen toward the floor as much as you can.

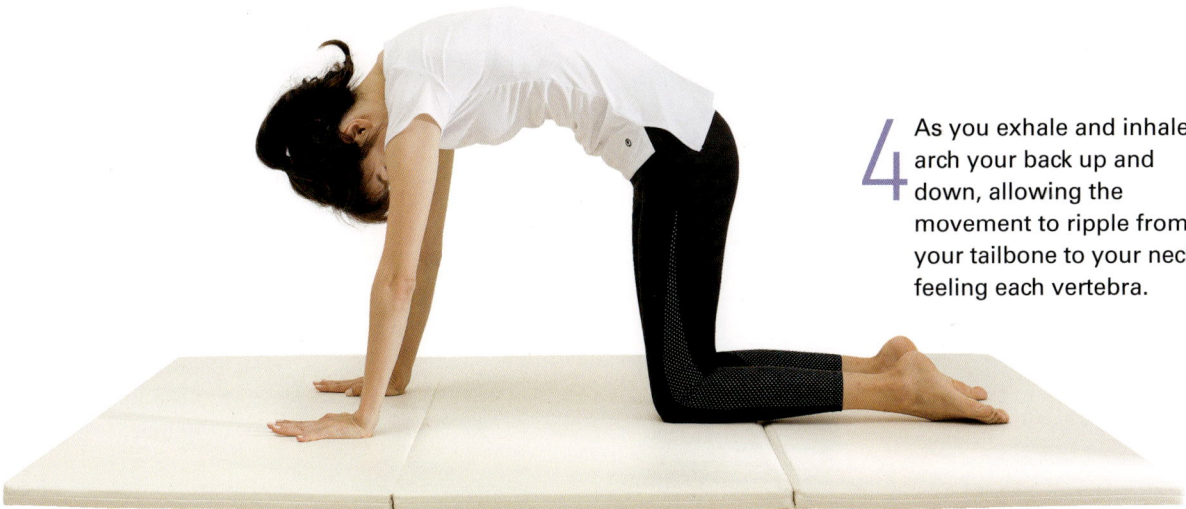

4 As you exhale and inhale, arch your back up and down, allowing the movement to ripple from your tailbone to your neck, feeling each vertebra.

* Repeat the movement eight times for three sets.

Tip

If you are familiar with the cat-cow yoga pose, you may notice that it's hard to maintain the steady speed because you might lift your spine up and down without being fully aware of your movements. Focus on rolling one vertebra at a time.

Bird Dog

This exercise can improve balance and strengthen the muscles throughout the body, especially hips and deltoids.

All Fours 2

1 Start in the all-fours position and inhale to begin.

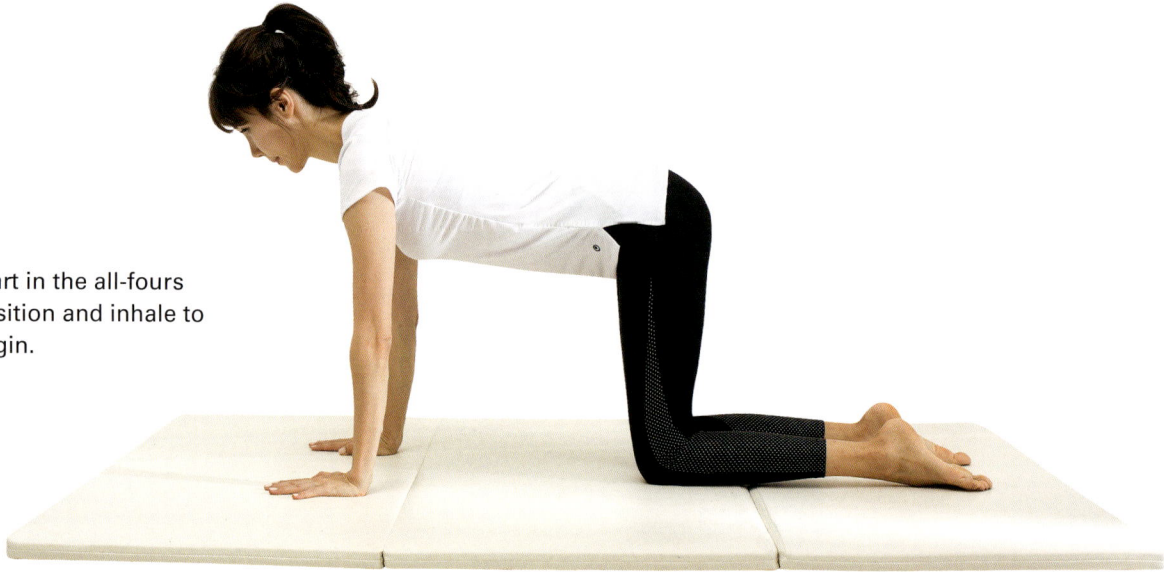

2 Extend your left leg back as you exhale.

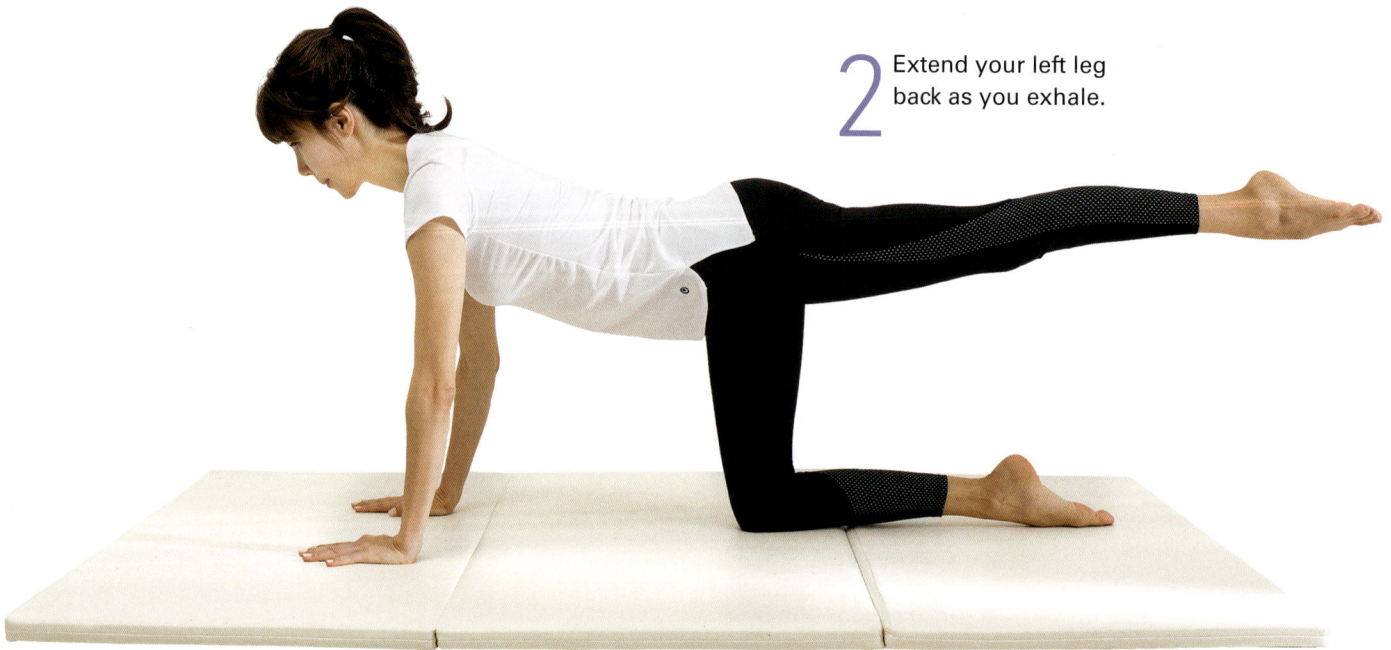

76

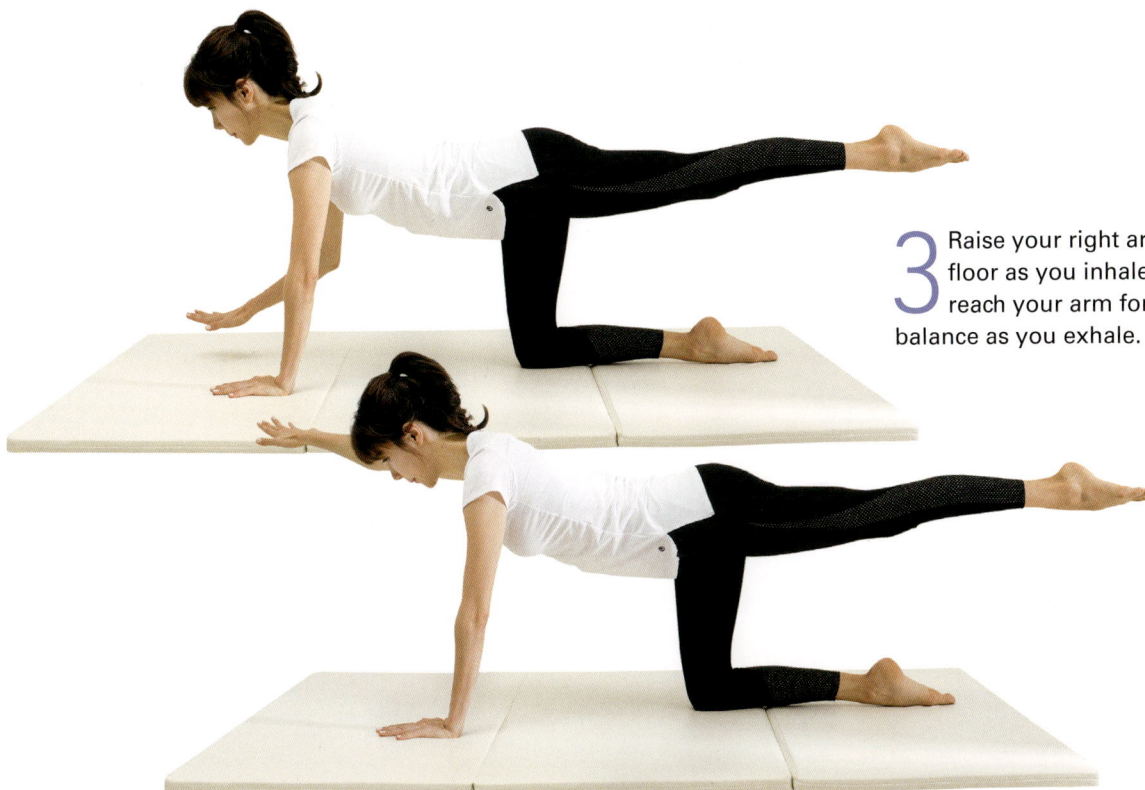

3 Raise your right arm off the floor as you inhale, then reach your arm forward to balance as you exhale.

4 Return to the starting position as you inhale. Repeat on the other side.

* Extend one leg and raise the opposite arm, then alternate on other side. Repeat for eight sets.

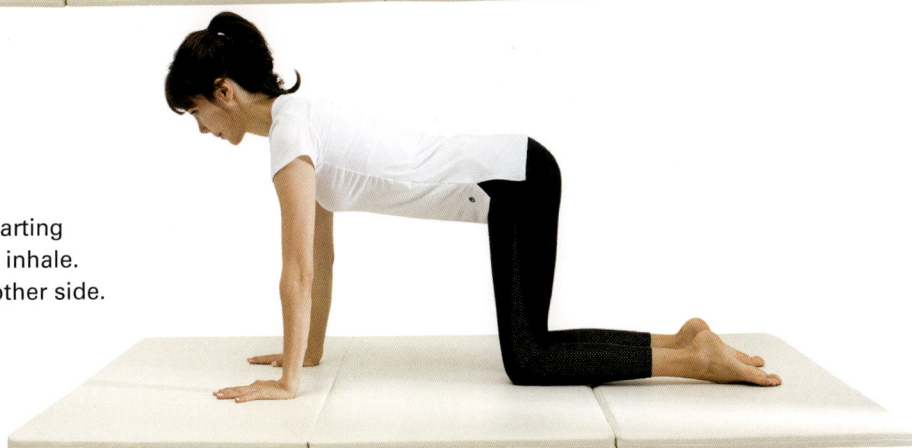

─ Tip ─

Connect each movement smoothly. Stretch one leg back and the opposite arm forward, then return to the starting position. Remember to elongate your arms and legs rather than just raise them up high.

Leg Kick-Back

This exercise can tone the hips and thighs, reduce lower body fat, and sculpt a strong, well-defined posterior.

1 Start in the all-fours position and inhale to begin.

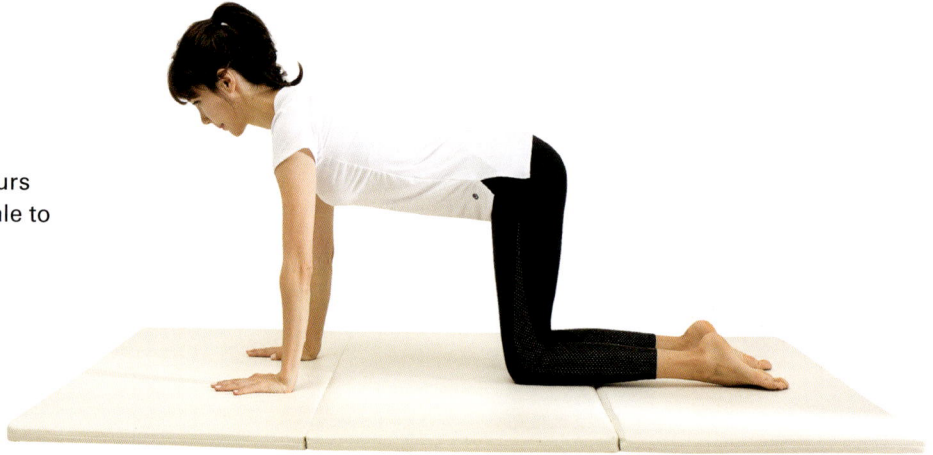

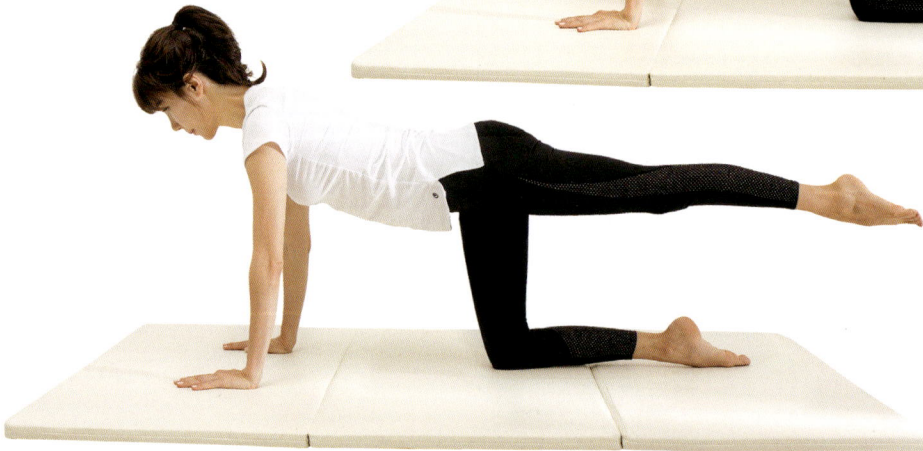

2 Extend your left leg back as you exhale.

3 Bring the left leg in toward the chest as you inhale, then extend the leg back as you exhale.

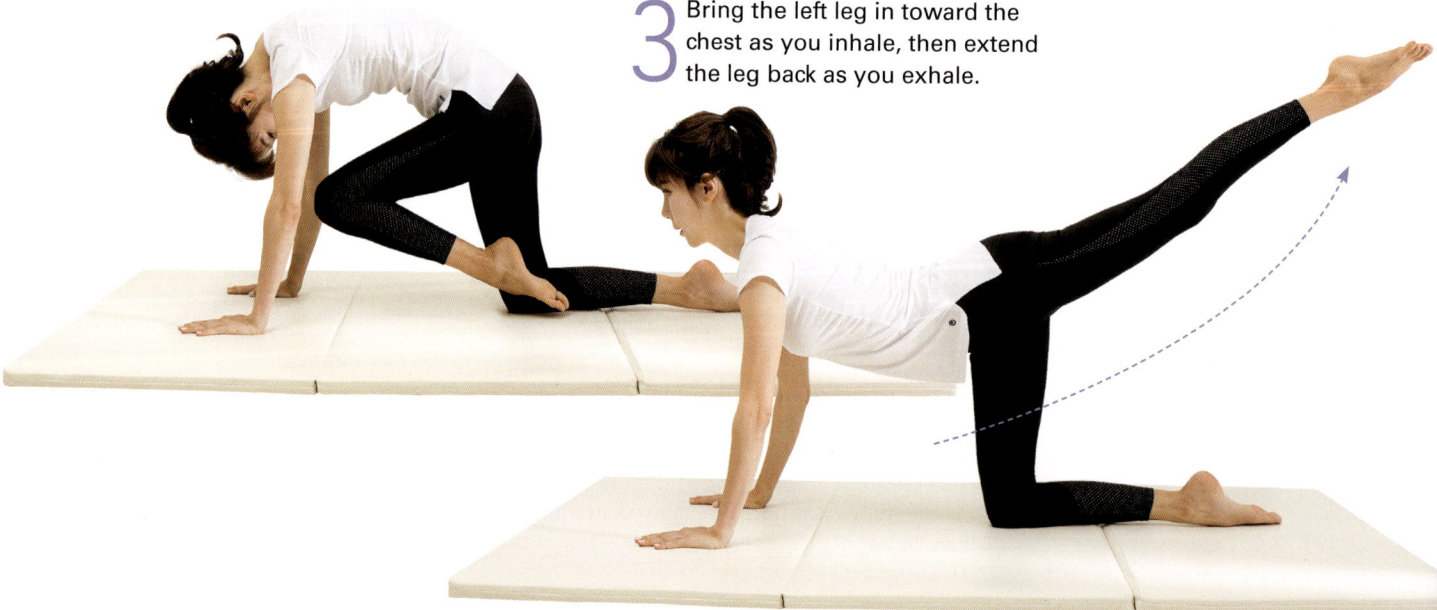

4 Lower the leg as you inhale, and raise the leg as you exhale. Repeat eight times.

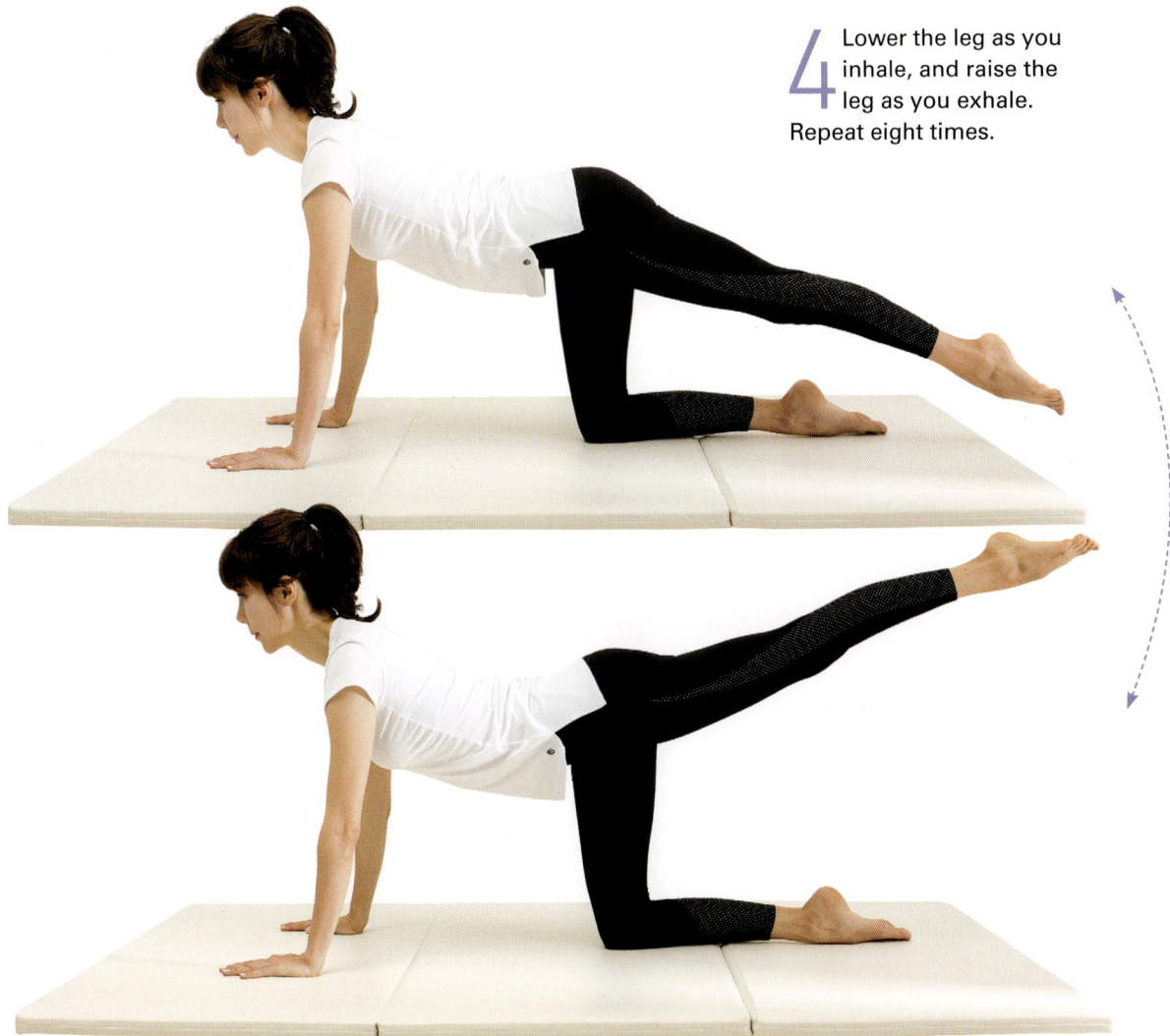

* Repeat three sets of movement 4 starting from your leg raised.

— Tip —

It's easy to lose your core balance while practicing this movement. Focus more on your hip and thigh muscles rather than kicking high. Keep your core tight and balanced as you raise your legs.

Lunge Stretching

This exercise helps correct pelvic and spinal misalignment caused by poor habits. It will help you to build a strong and supple spine and increase the blood circulation.

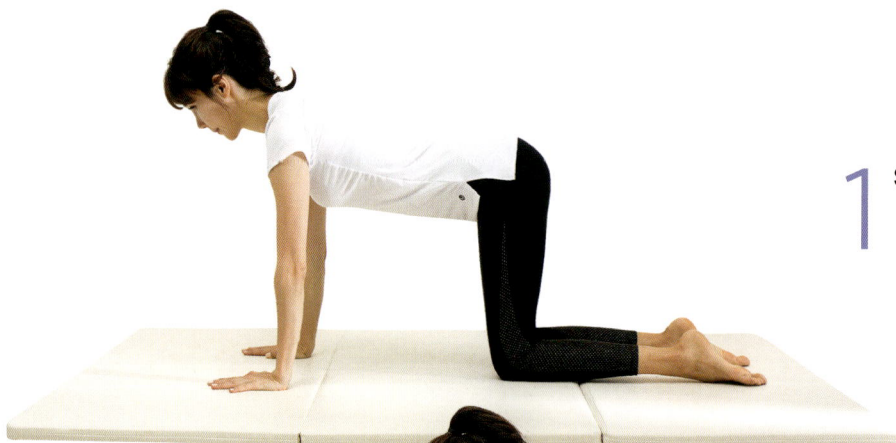

1 Start in the all-fours position.

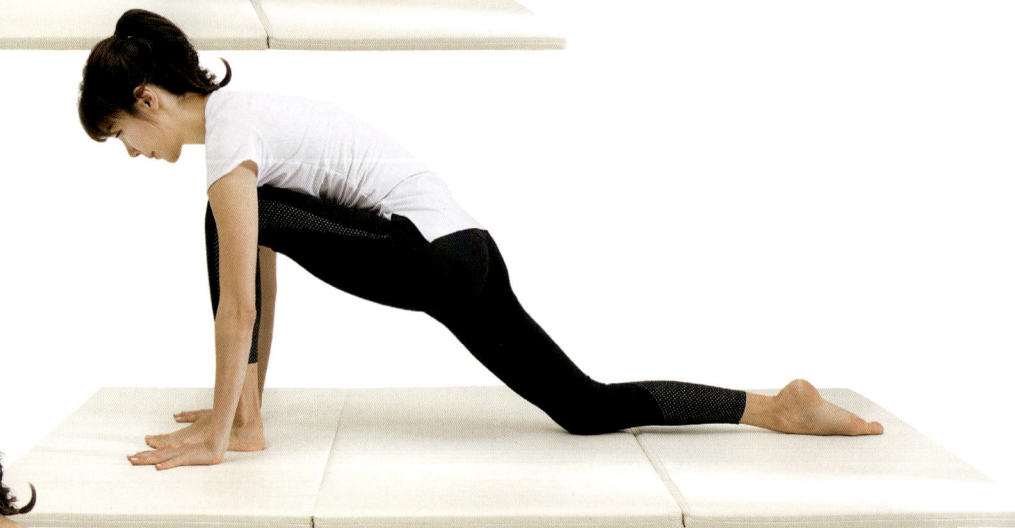

2 Take a big step with your left foot as you inhale, and stretch your arms to the floor while keeping your balance.

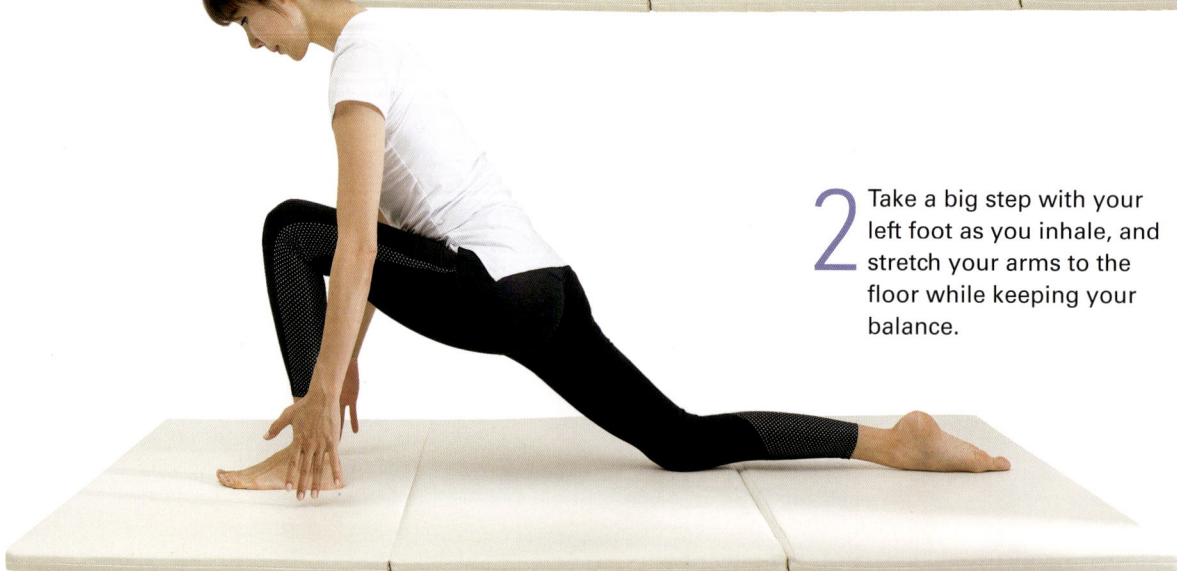

3 Reach both arms up as you exhale and bring your torso forward.

4 Reach your arms to the side and straighten your left knee as you inhale to return to the neutral position.

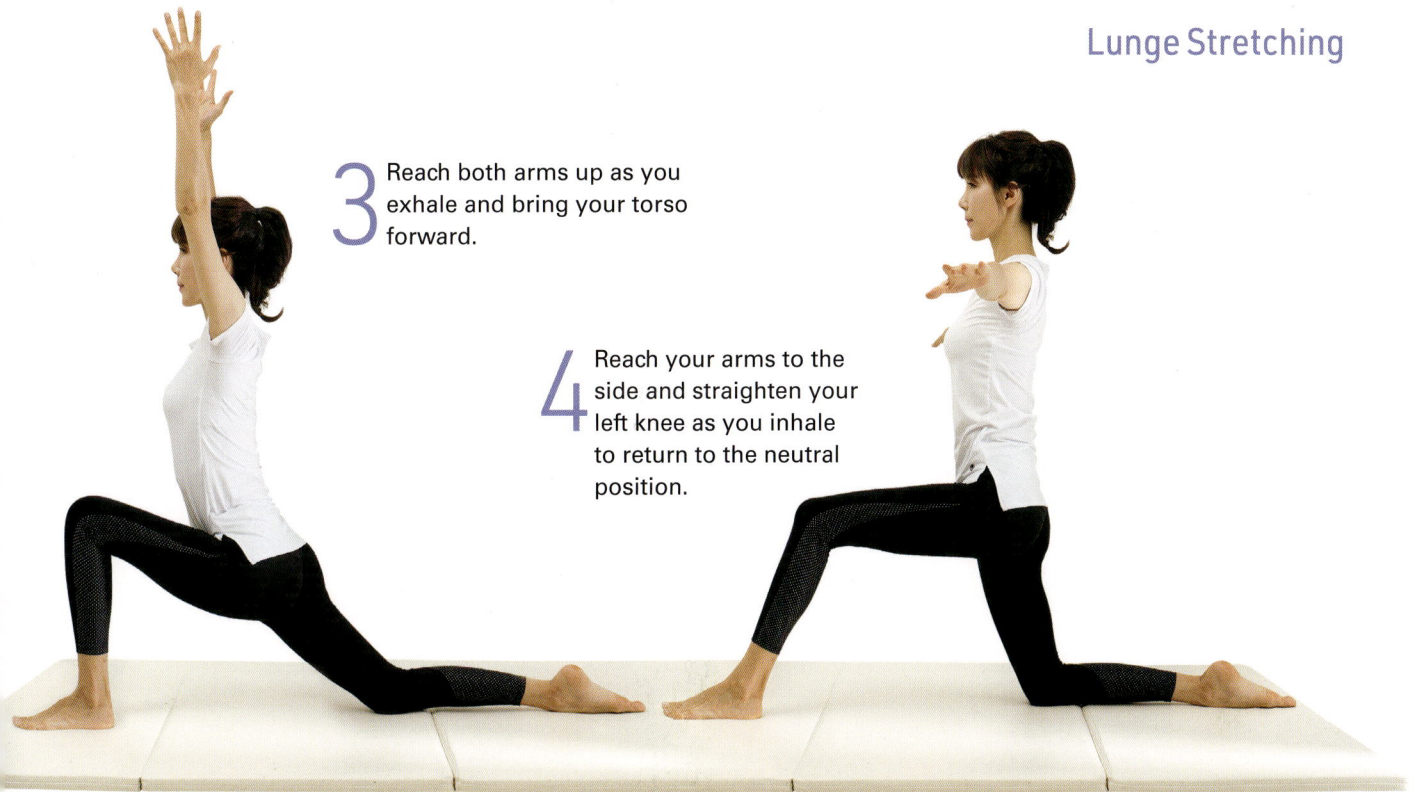

5 Reach your arms up and bring your torso forward as you inhale, then stretch your arms to the side and bring your torso back as you exhale.

* Repeat eight times on each side.

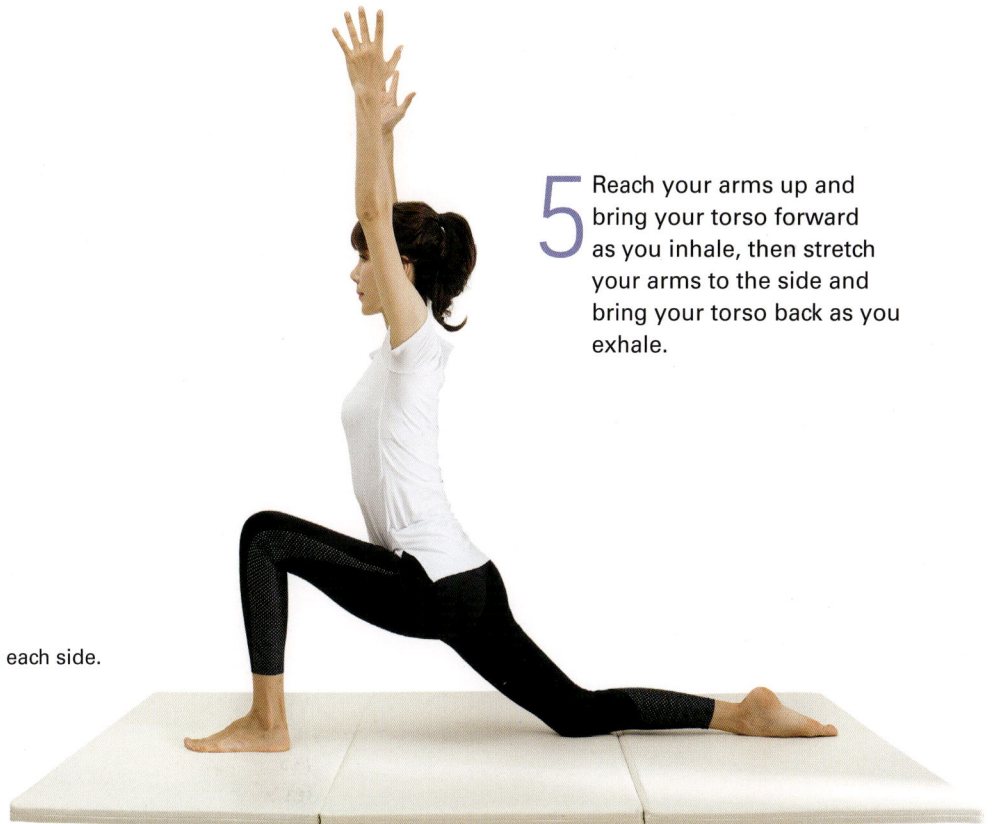

Tip

If you lack flexibility, keeping your knees stacked over your ankle when you stretch can be challenging. Adjust your step length to help align the knees and maintain the correct posture.

Leg Pull–Front

This exercise helps build a fit, balanced body by improving stability, control, and posture. You can modify the movement to suit your level.

All Fours
5

2 Start in the all-fours position.

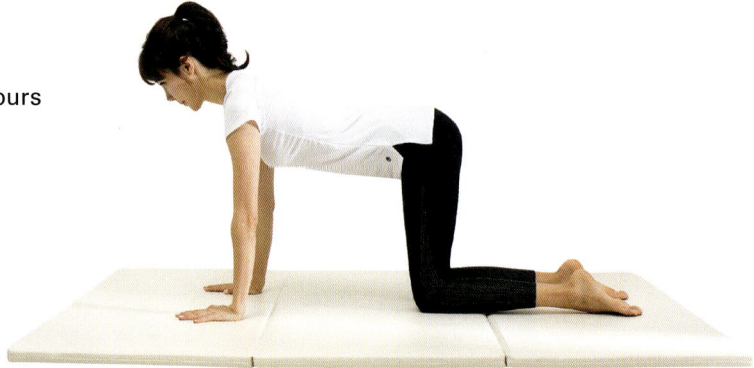

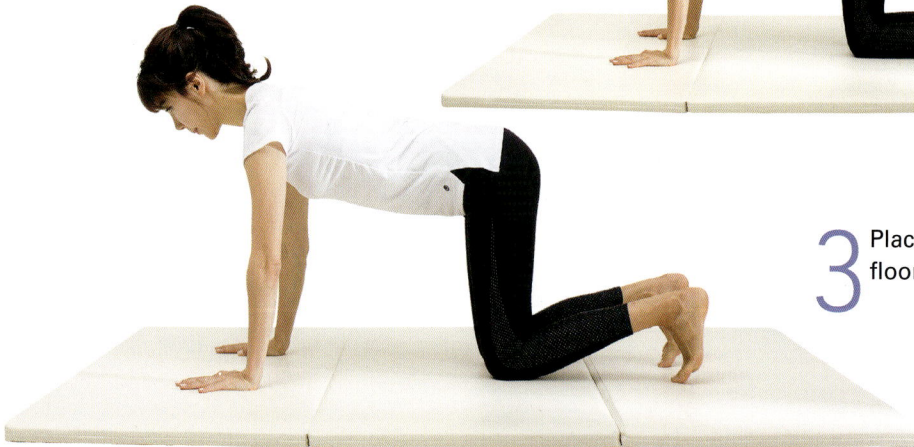

3 Place your toes on the floor and inhale to begin.

4 First stretch your left leg and then your right as you inhale. Create a long, diagonal line from head to toe.

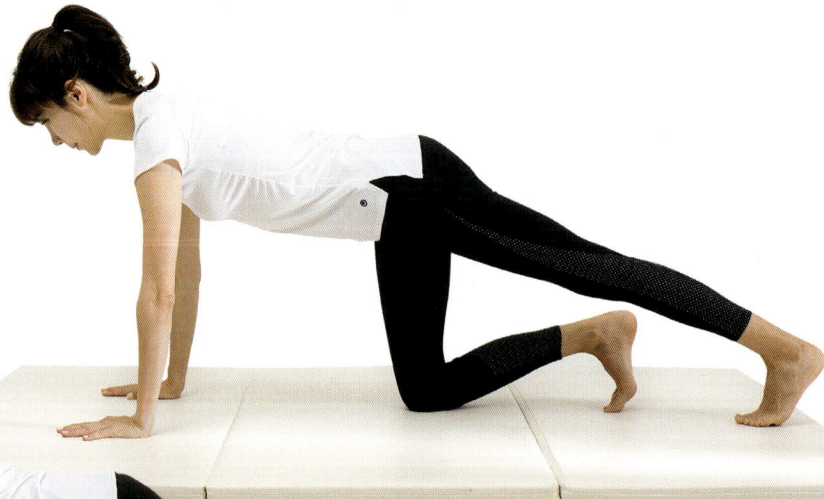

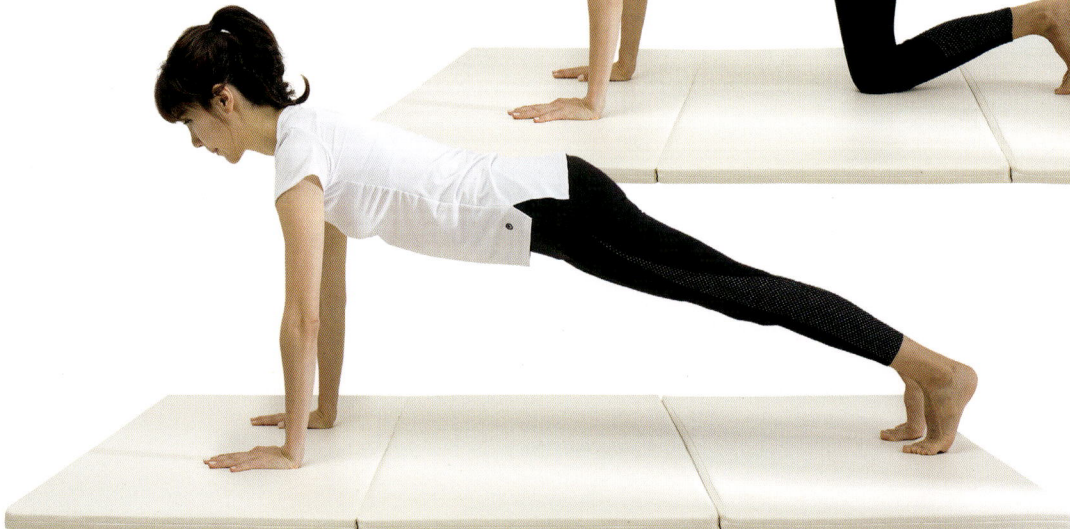

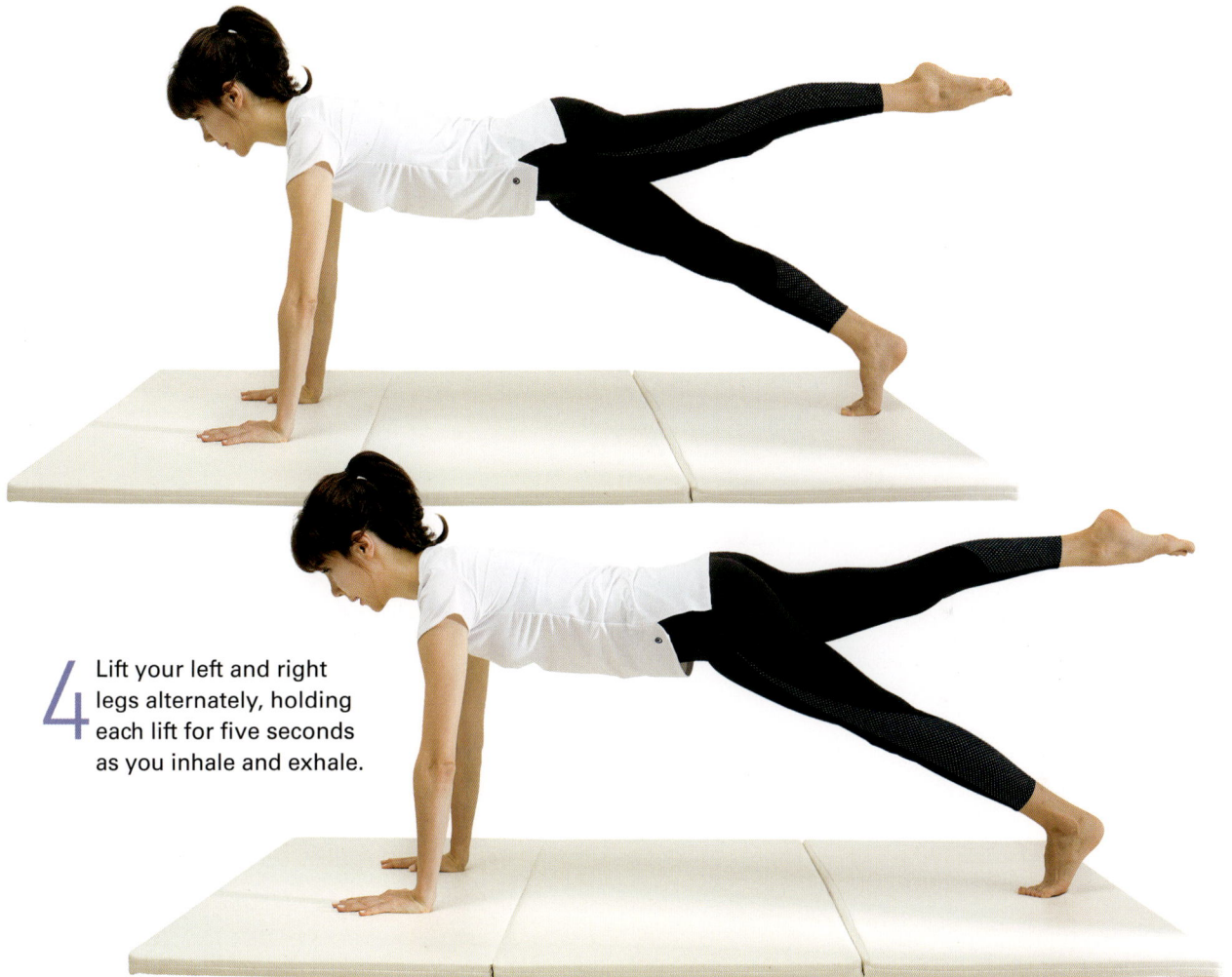

4 Lift your left and right legs alternately, holding each lift for five seconds as you inhale and exhale.

* Repeat movement 4 eight times for three sets.

— Tip —

It's important to keep your arms and spine straight and your core tightened. If your core weakens, your torso might lower and your arms and legs might overstrain, which can injure your shoulders or back. Focus on your breathing and your core to maintain the correct posture.

Supine

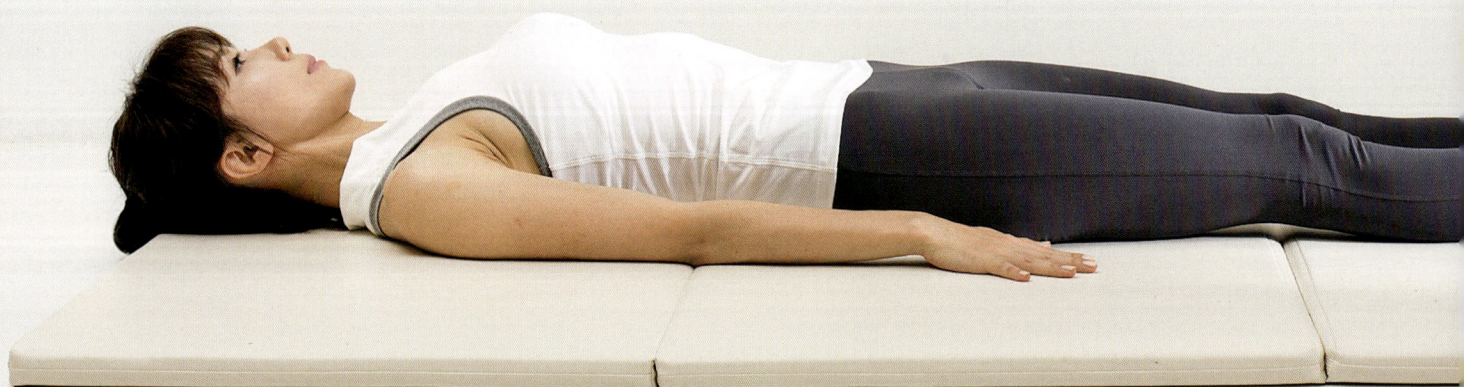

Neutral Posture

Many Pilates exercises begin in the supine position. Done correctly, this position requires core engagement, which can strengthen the abdominal and back muscles and realign and condition the body. Maintain the natural curve of the spine so you don't overstrain the back.

Correct Posture ✓

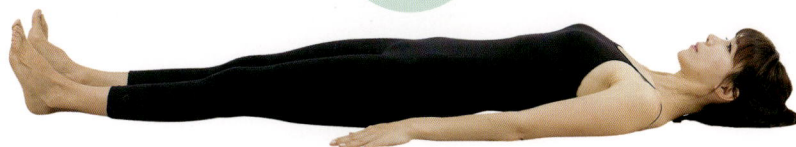

Incorrect Posture ✗

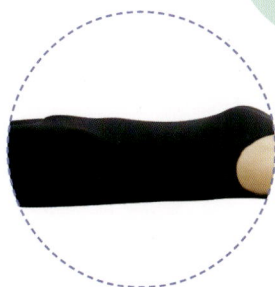

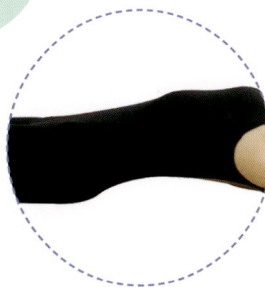

Leg Sliding

This exercise tones the abdominal muscles and enhances the ability to control the core and lower body.

1 Lie on your back with your knees bent. Place both hands on your lower abdomen and contract your abdomen to begin.

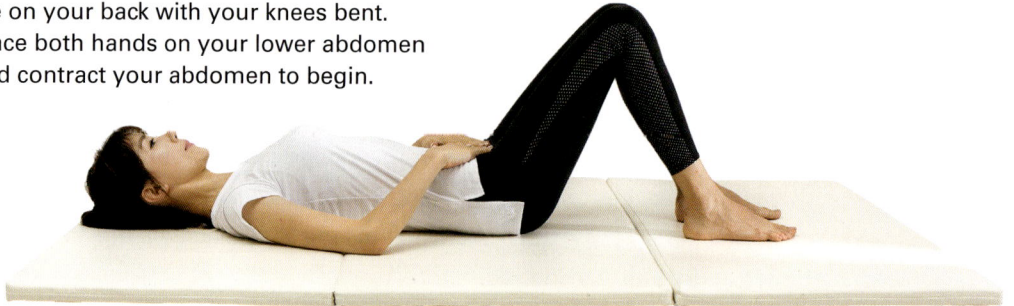

2 Extend your right leg as you exhale.

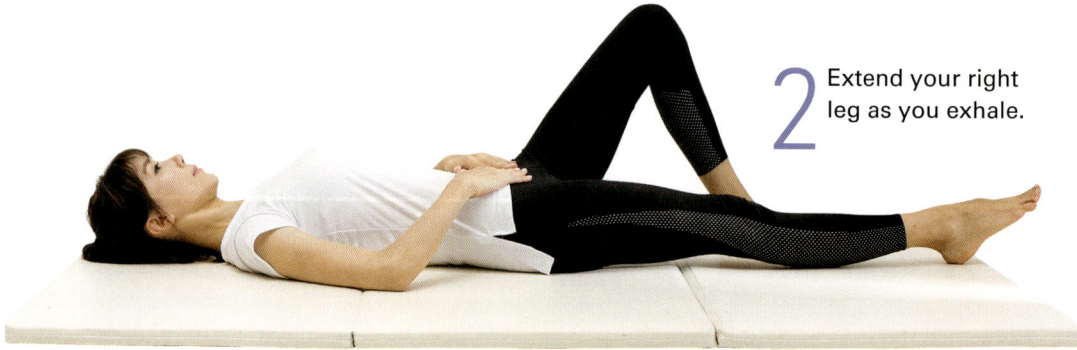

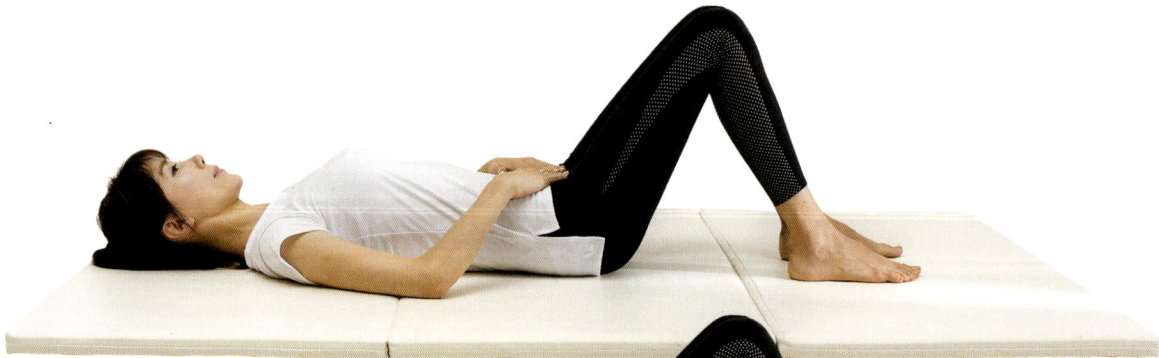

3 Return to the starting position and extend your left leg.

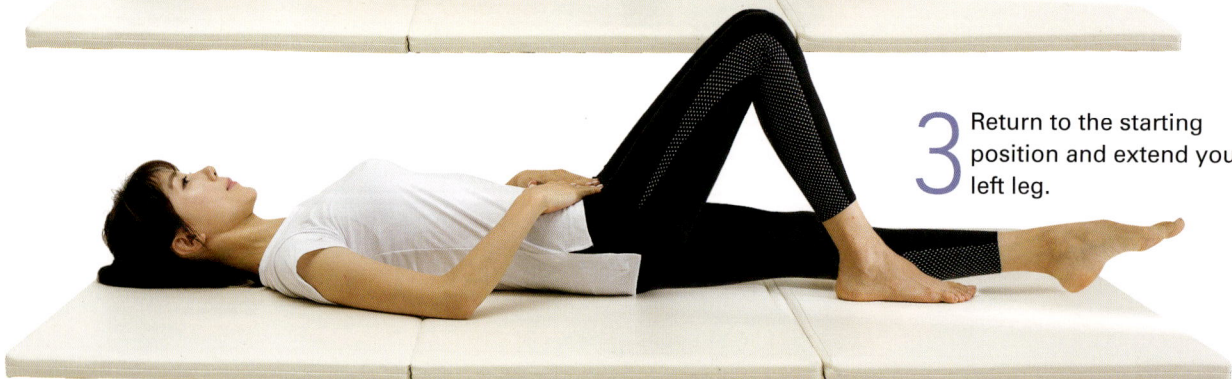

*Alternate the leg for eight times.

86

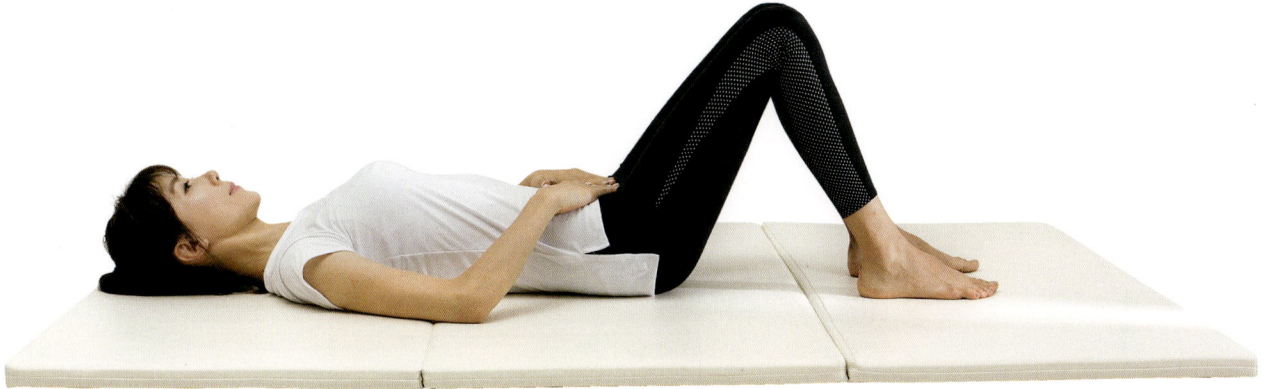

4 Bend your knees to return to the starting position and slide both legs down the floor as you exhale. Return to the starting position as you inhale.

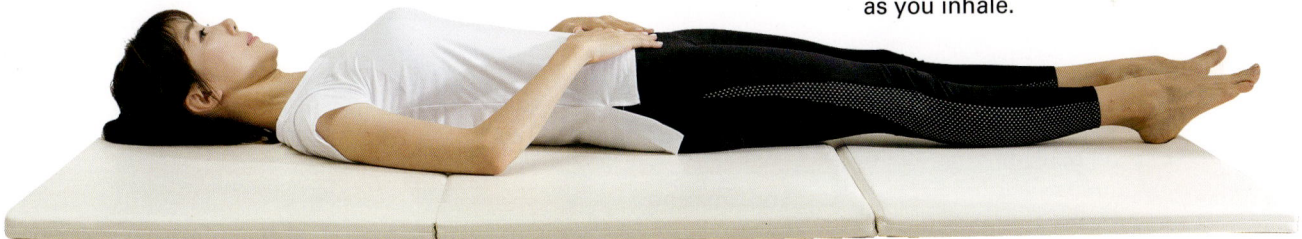

* Repeat eight sets of movements 2 to 4.

— Tip —

If you overstrain your body and focus solely on contracting your abdomen, you may create unnecessary tension. Instead, breathe in a steady rhythm and focus on your core.

One-Leg Stretch

This core-focused exercise strengthens the pelvic region and waist while targeting the lower abdomen and legs. Repeatedly stretching and drawing in the hip joint helps tone the body.

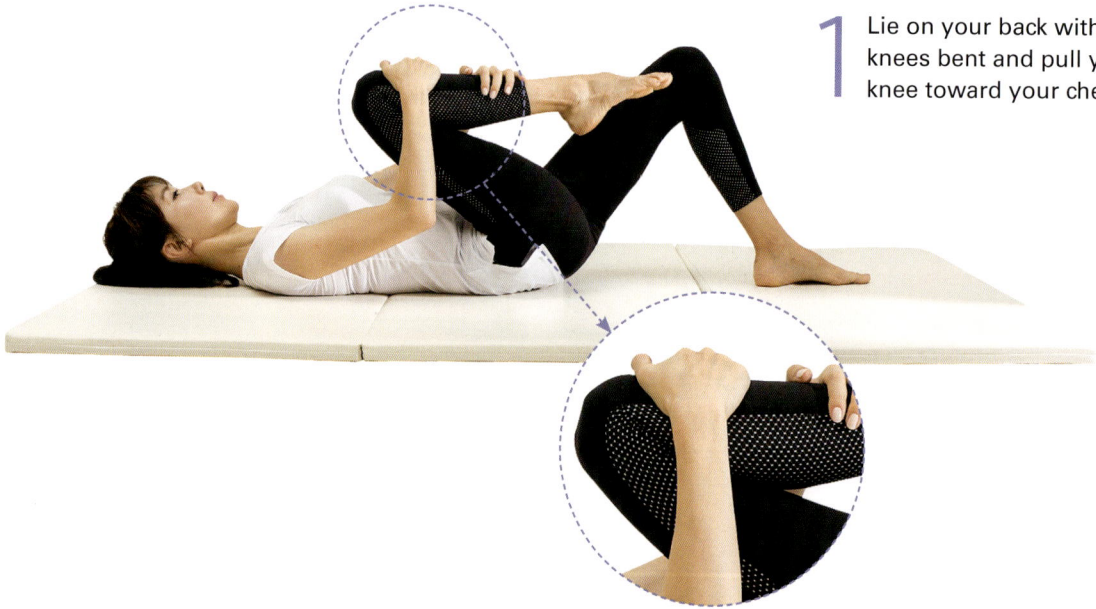

1 Lie on your back with your knees bent and pull your right knee toward your chest.

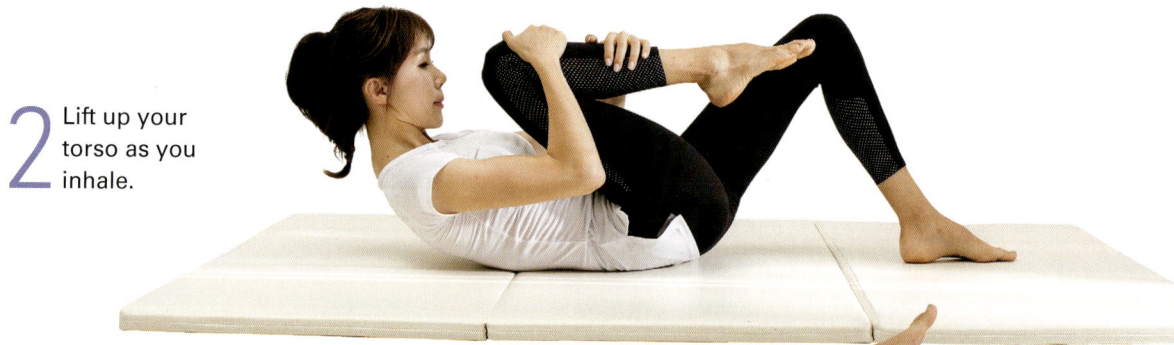

2 Lift up your torso as you inhale.

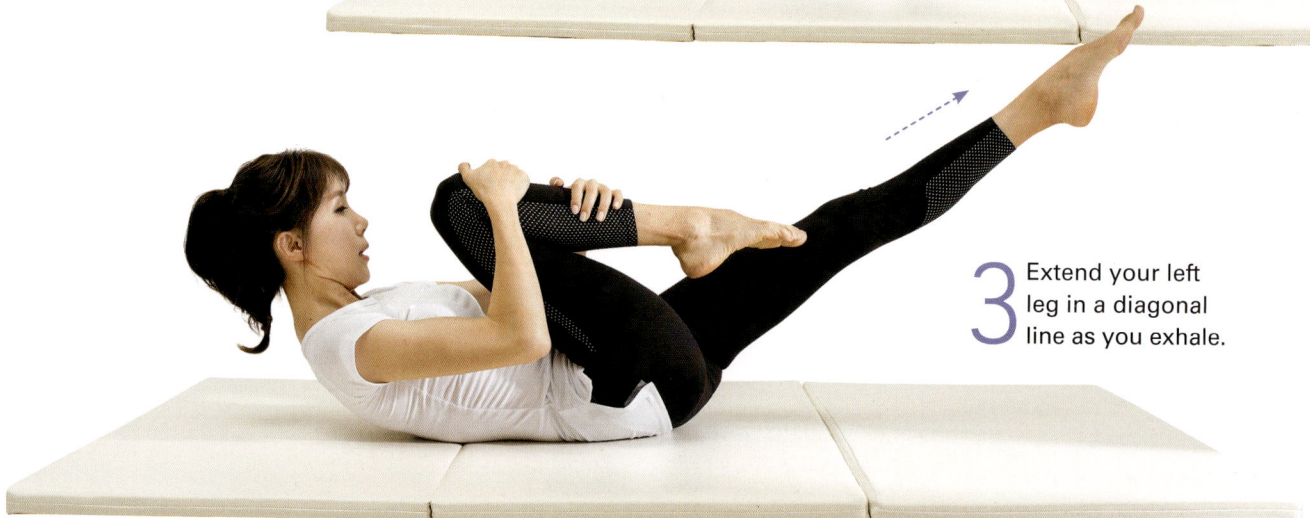

3 Extend your left leg in a diagonal line as you exhale.

88

4 Lift up your torso until your shoulders are off the ground. Maintain the posture.

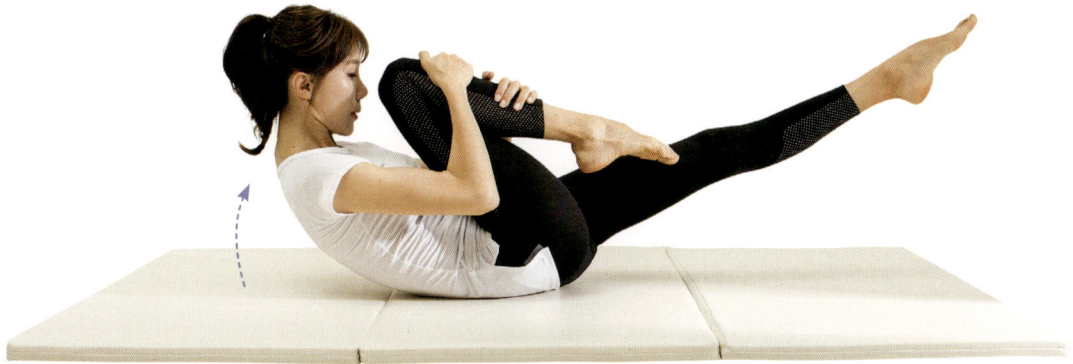

5 Alternate legs while breathing rhythmically.

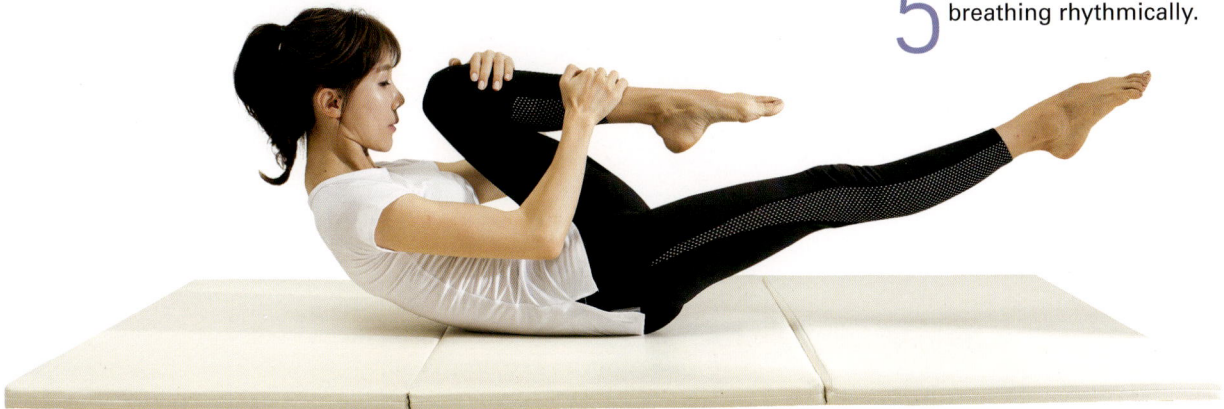

* Repeat eight times on each leg for three sets.

Tip

If you lack flexibility in the hip joints or feel back pain, take it more slowly and don't overstrain your body. Posing in a perfect posture doesn't always result in perfection. You have to acknowledge your capability and practice regularly to make progress.

The Hundred

This Pilates classic uses simple, repetitive movement to warm up the entire body and activate the core muscles. It enhances stability and increases circulation.

1 Lie on your back comfortably and reach your arms overhead as you inhale.

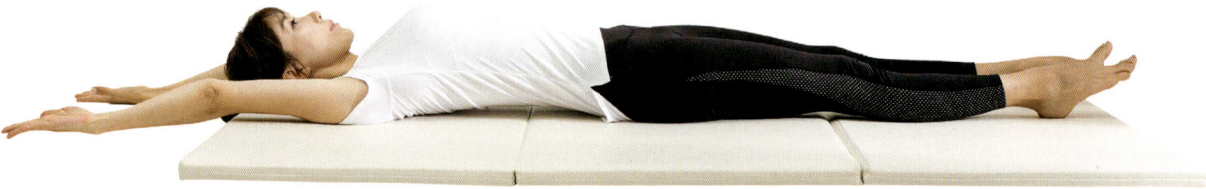

2 Lift up your torso and draw it slightly forward as you exhale.

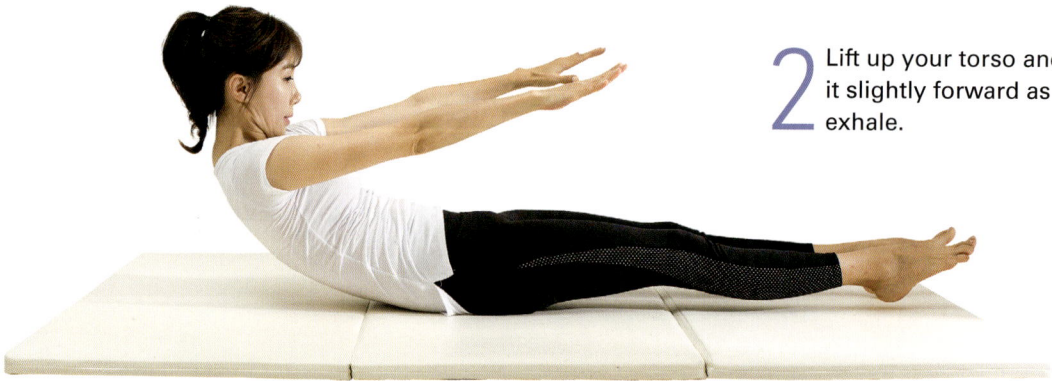

3 Raise both legs and extend them. As you inhale and exhale, pump your arms up and down with small, controlled movements for 100 counts.

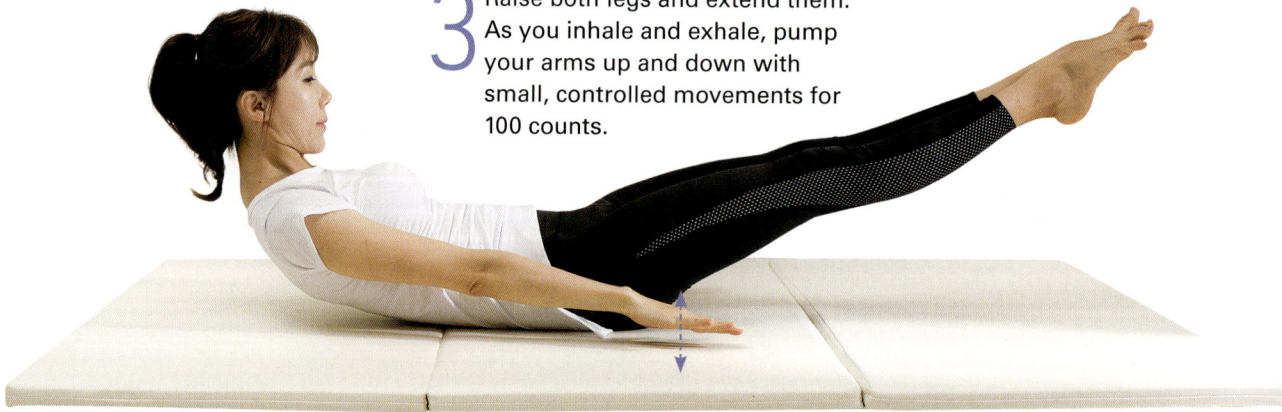

* Pump your arms five times as you inhale, then another five times as you exhale. Start with fewer repetitions, then gradually progress to 100.

Variation

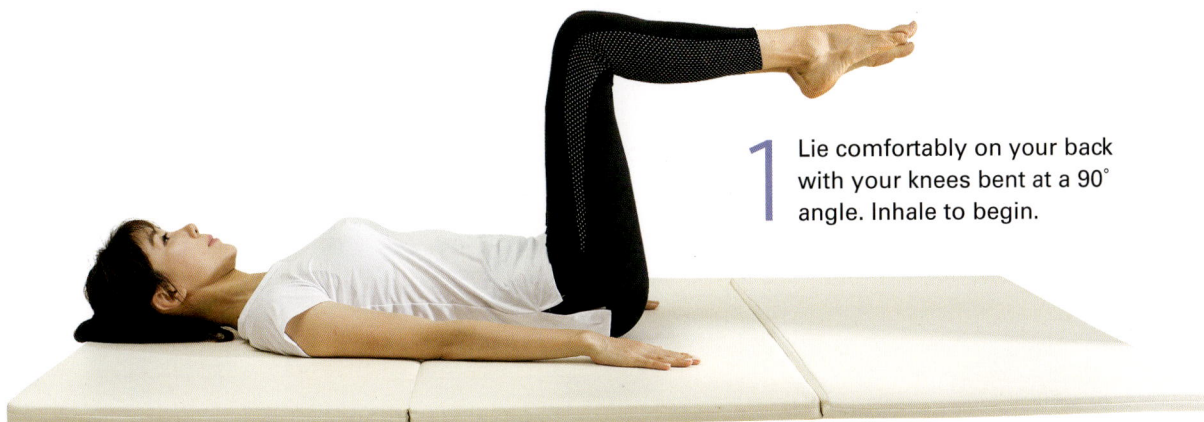

1 Lie comfortably on your back with your knees bent at a 90° angle. Inhale to begin.

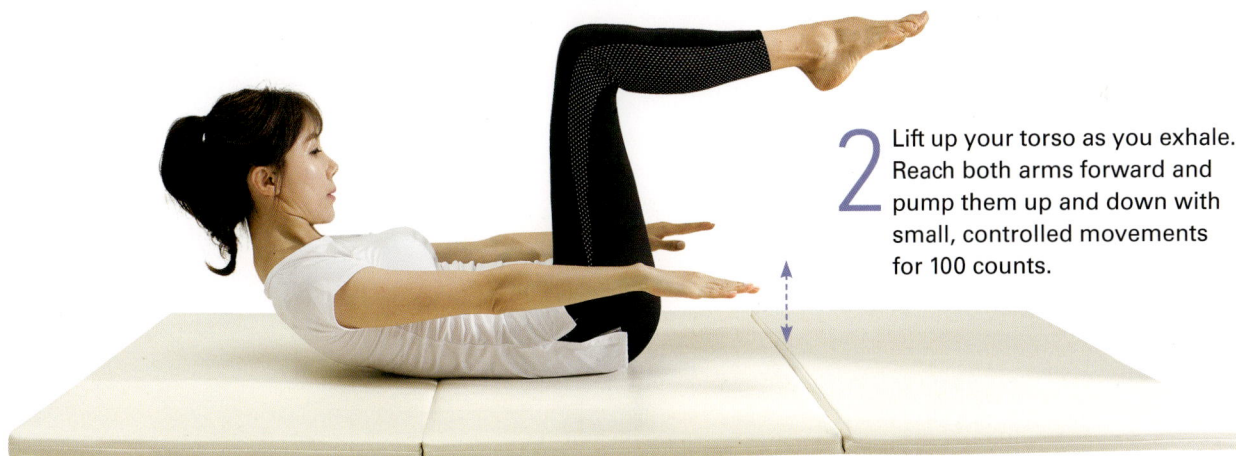

2 Lift up your torso as you exhale. Reach both arms forward and pump them up and down with small, controlled movements for 100 counts.

* It's easier to practice with your knees bent.

— Tip —

The Hundred is a foundational Pilates exercise that can be adapted to suit different fitness levels. Start with the basic version and gradually progress to more advanced variations as you improve.

Roll-Up

Articulating movement through each vertebra improves spinal alignment. This exercise also enhances core stability and increases flexibility.

1 Lie flat on your back and bring your legs together with your arms stretched overhead. Inhale to begin.

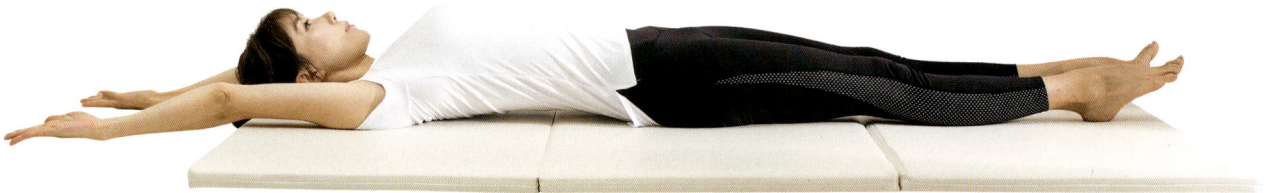

2 Lift up your torso with your arms reaching forward as you exhale.

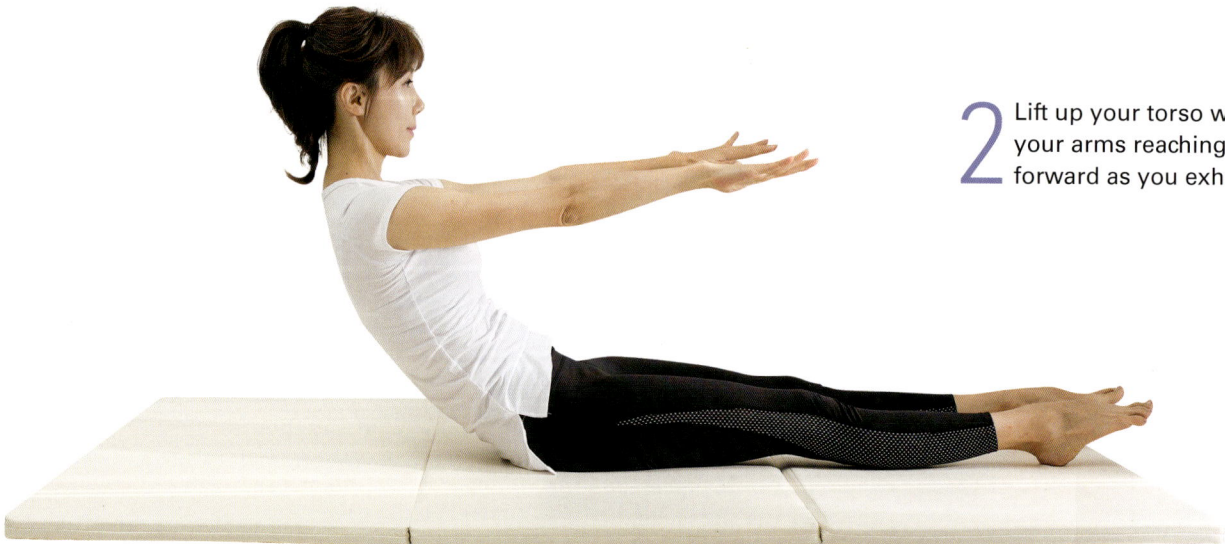

3 Round your spine to bend forward as you inhale.

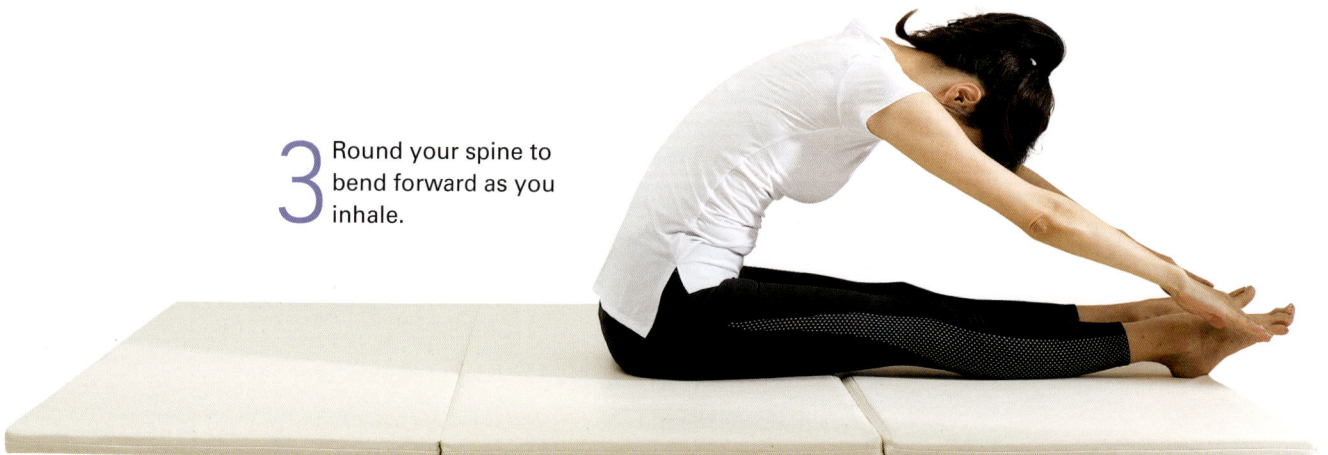

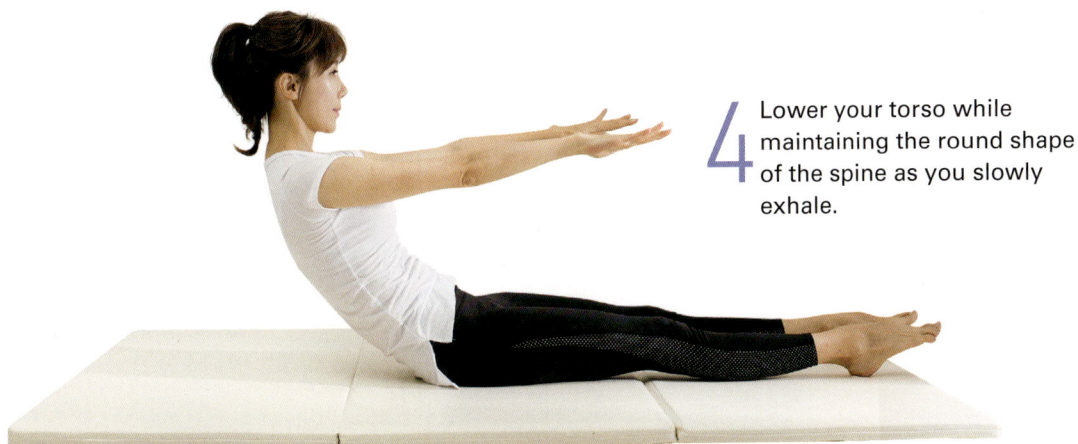

4 Lower your torso while maintaining the round shape of the spine as you slowly exhale.

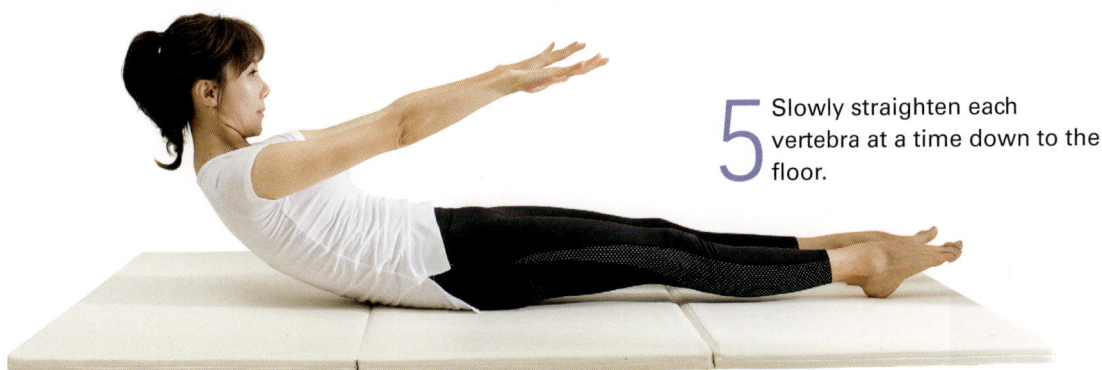

5 Slowly straighten each vertebra at a time down to the floor.

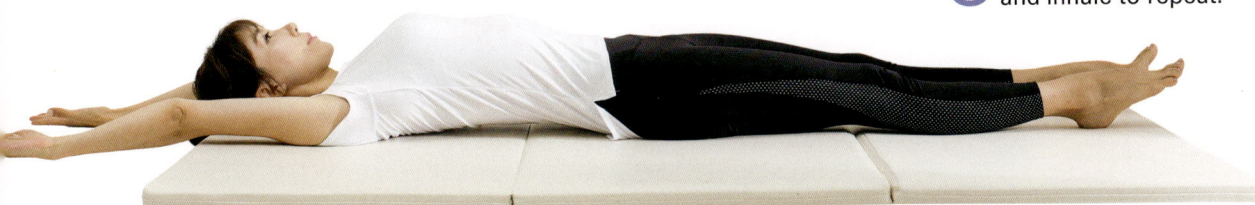

6 When you are flat on the floor, stretch your arms overhead and inhale to repeat.

* Repeat three times at a slow pace.

― Tip ―

You may not be perfect from the start. If you lack strength in your legs or abdomen, practice the "Single Leg Roll-Up" (p. 122). You can use a towel instead of the ring.

Roll-Over

This exercise helps correct spinal alignment, improve blood circulation, and increase back flexibility. It may also help relieve symptoms of sciatica.

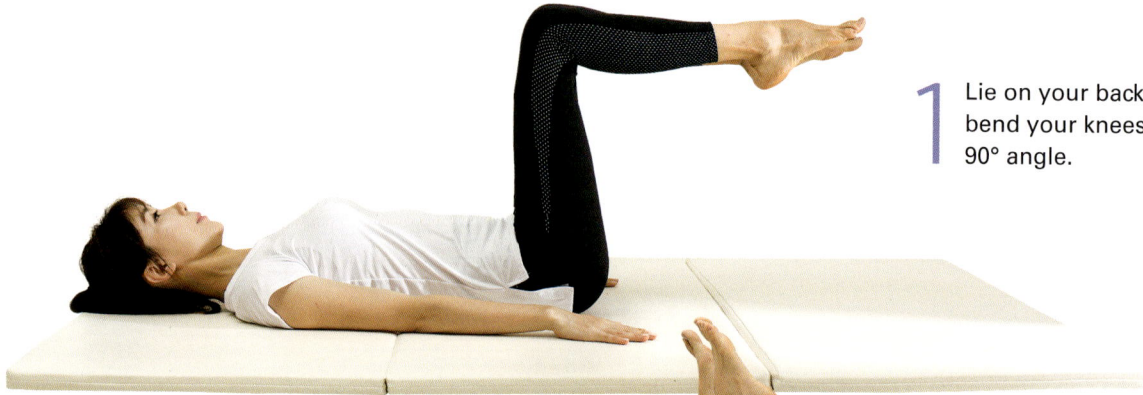

1 Lie on your back and bend your knees to a 90° angle.

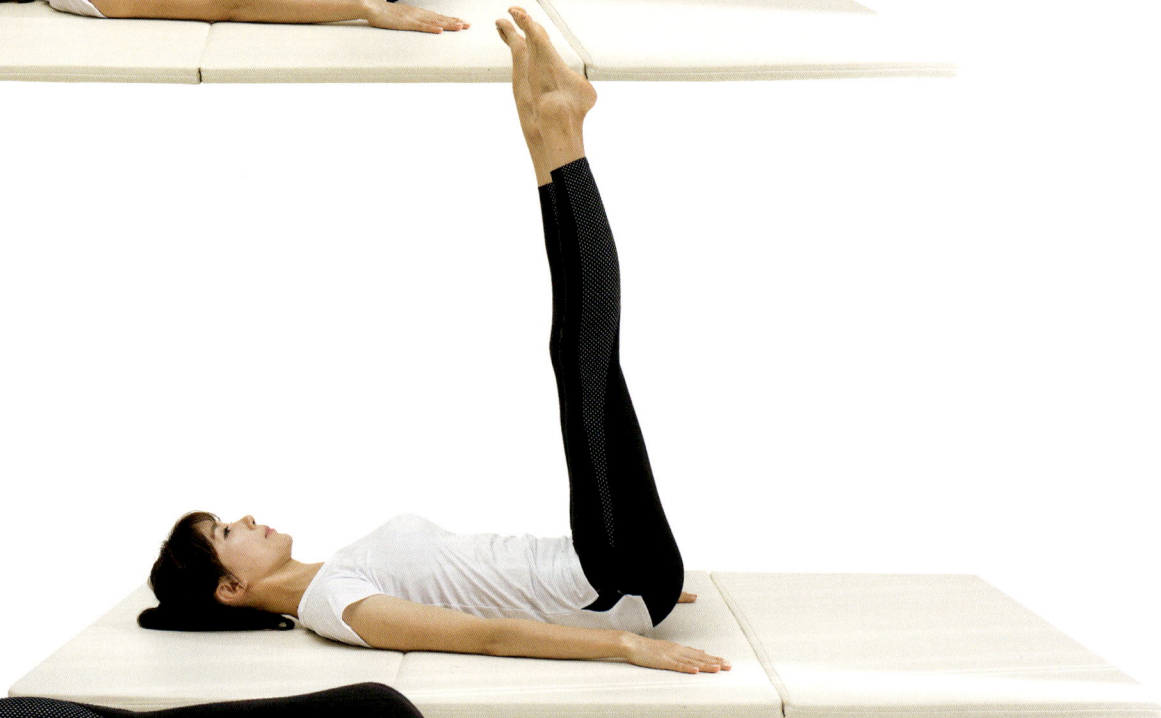

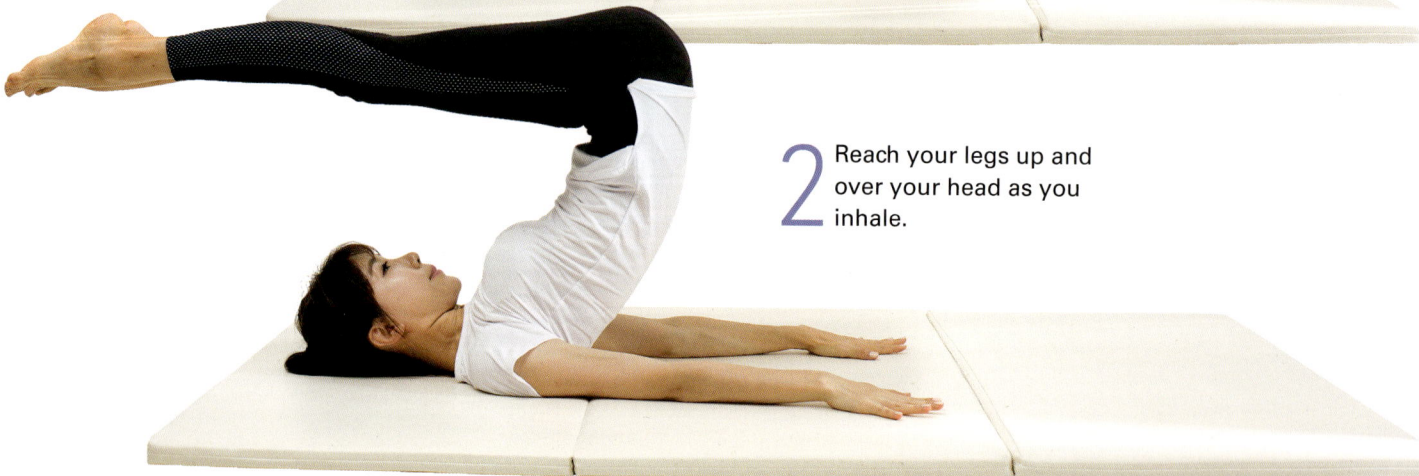

2 Reach your legs up and over your head as you inhale.

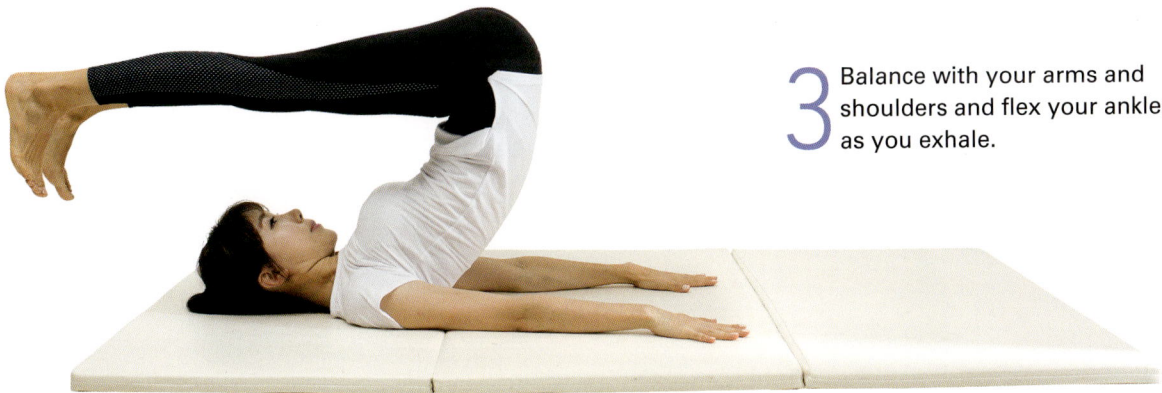

3 Balance with your arms and shoulders and flex your ankles as you exhale.

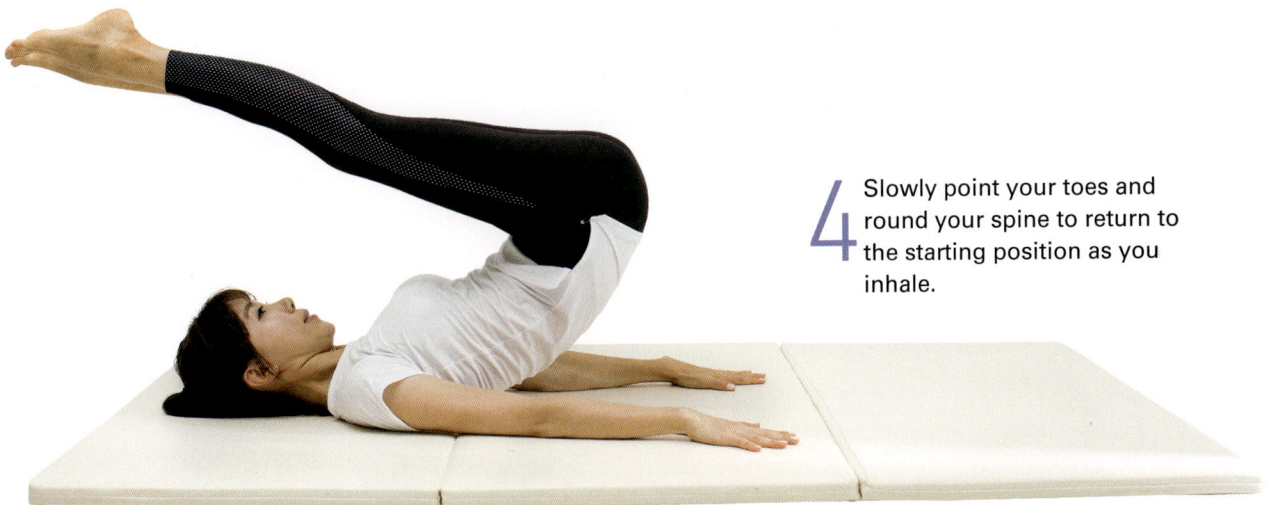

4 Slowly point your toes and round your spine to return to the starting position as you inhale.

* Repeat five times at a slow pace.

Tip

Make sure you do not bend your knees when you lift your legs up and down. Focus on articulating through each vertebra and support your neck and head to maintain balance and avoid straining your neck.

The Bicycle

This exercise promotes blood circulation in the lower body and improves core balance. It helps tone and slim the lower body and may relieve constipation.

1 Lie flat on your back and raise both legs in the air.

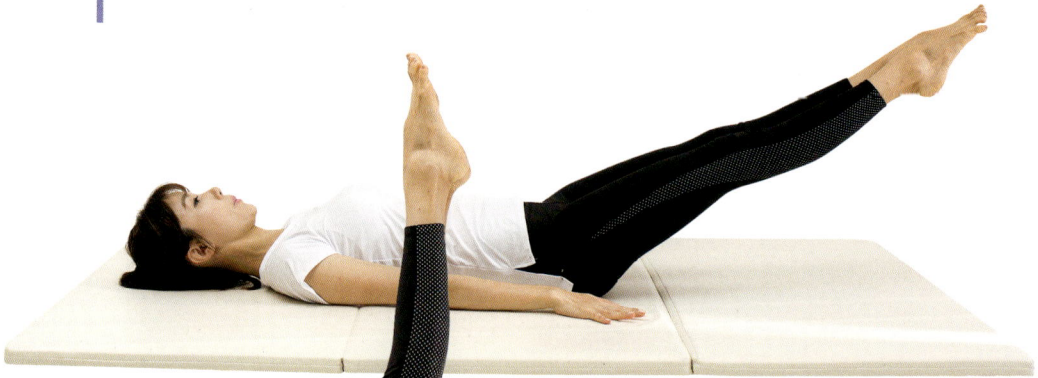

2 Lift up your torso as you inhale and support it with your arms to begin.

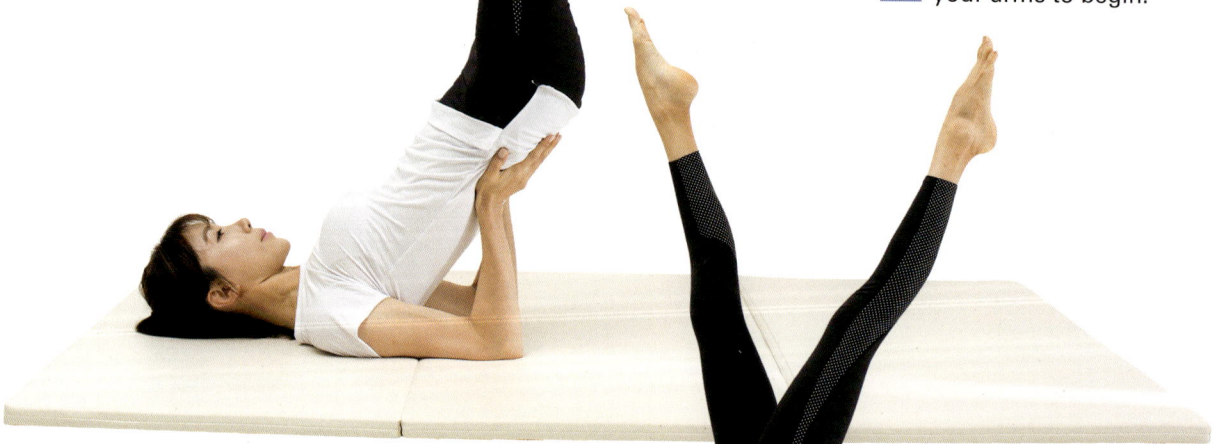

3 Cross your legs in the air while maintaining your balance as you exhale.

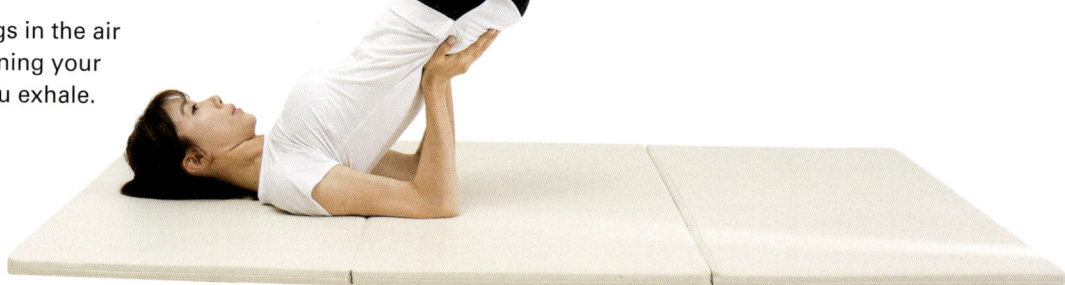

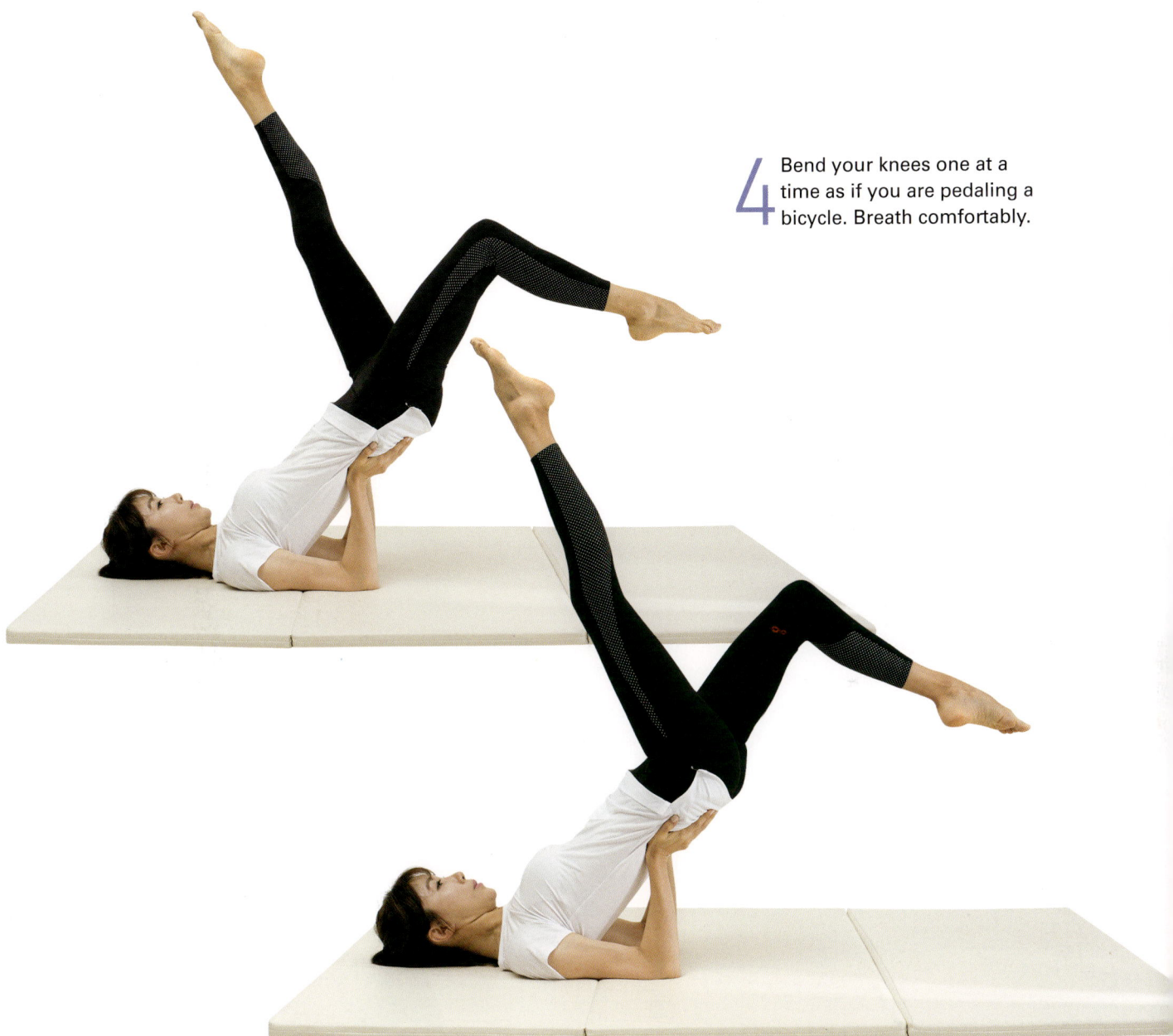

4 Bend your knees one at a time as if you are pedaling a bicycle. Breath comfortably.

* Repeat 10 times on each leg for two sets.

— Tip —

Begin the exercise only when your back feels firmly supported and balanced. Be careful not to move your head or torso, as this may cause injury.

Rolling Back

This exercise helps relax and align the spine by gently massaging it through a controlled rolling motion.

1 Sit with your knees bent and hold your shins with your arms.

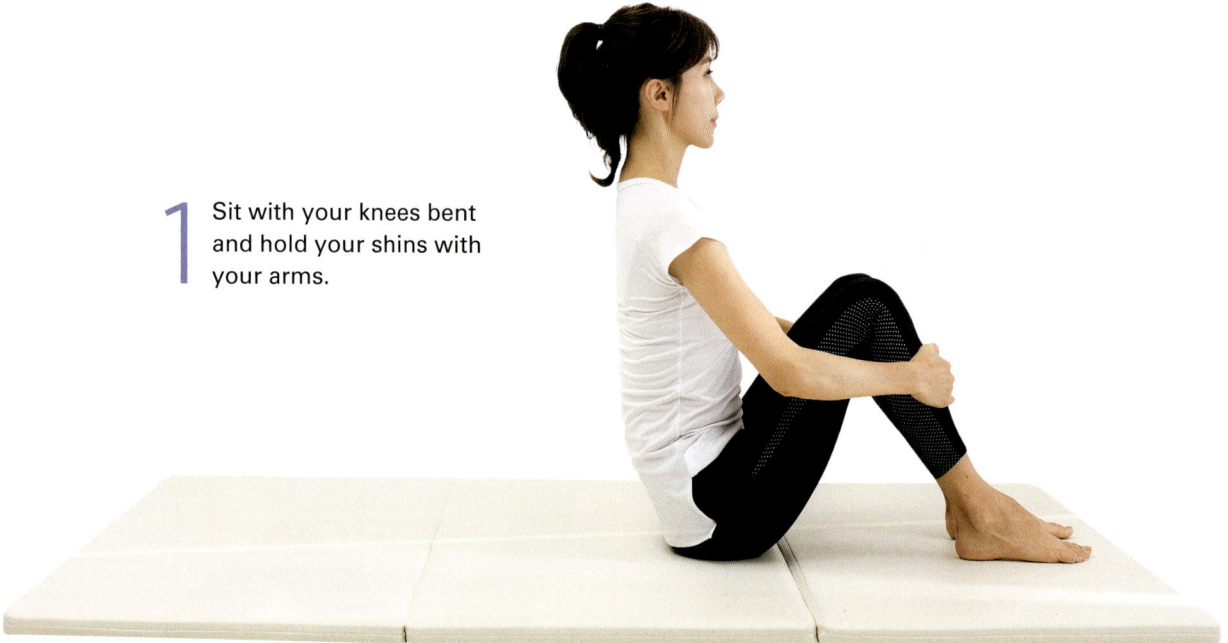

2 Round your back as you exhale, and lift both feet off the floor.

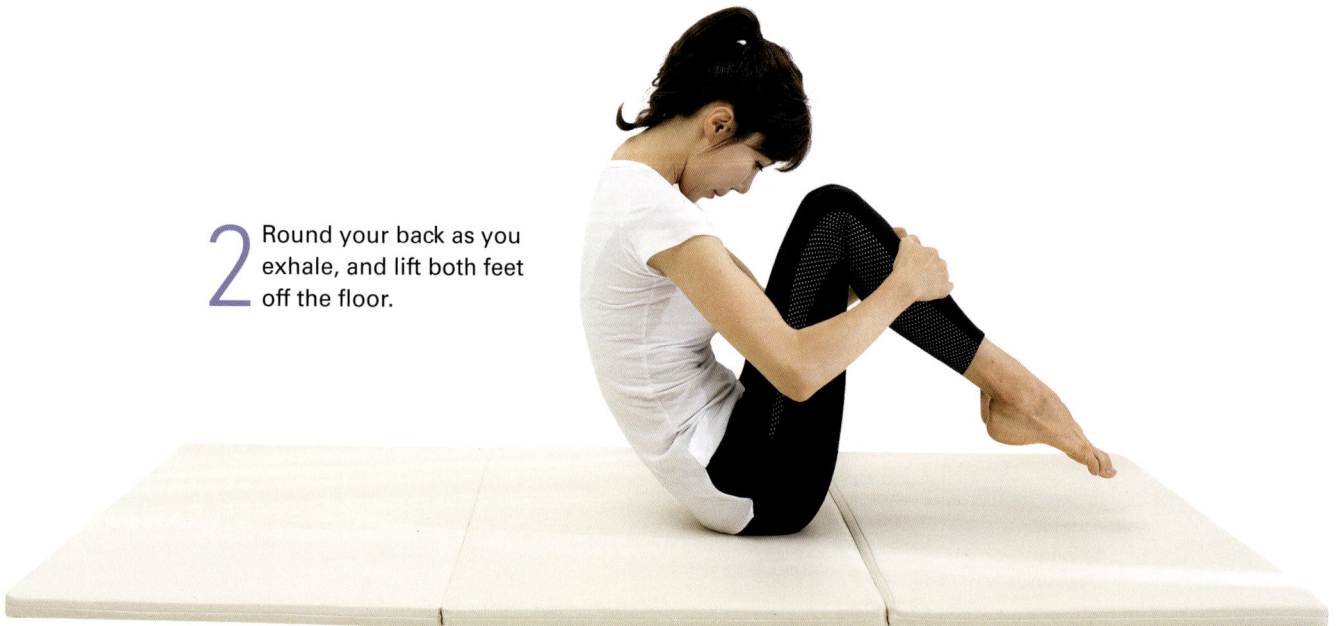

98

3 Roll back as you inhale.

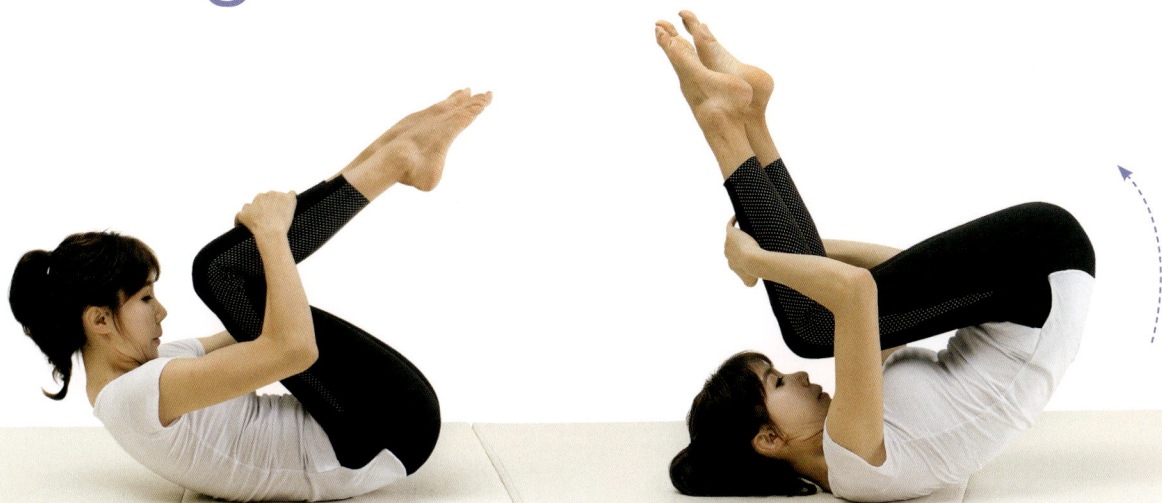

4 Return to the starting position as you exhale.

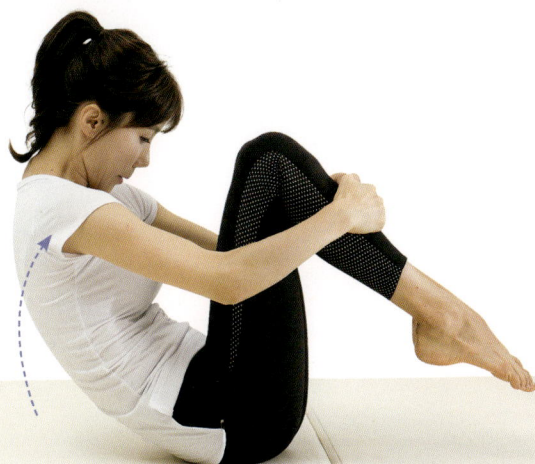

* Roll back and forth six times.

--- Tip ---

It's easier to roll if you hold the backs of your knees. As you progress with the movement, hold your shins, then your ankles, engaging the core fully to maintain control throughout the roll.

The Scissors

This exercise enhances blood circulation in the lower body and improves hamstring and hip flexibility. It will also tone and strengthen when practiced regularly.

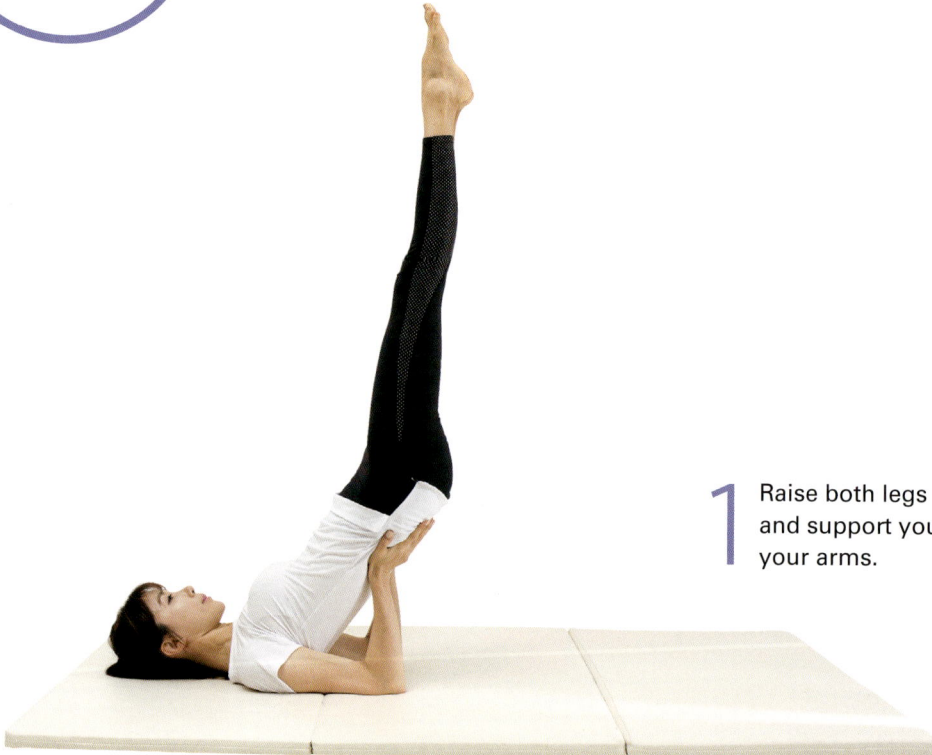

1 Raise both legs as you inhale, and support your torso with your arms.

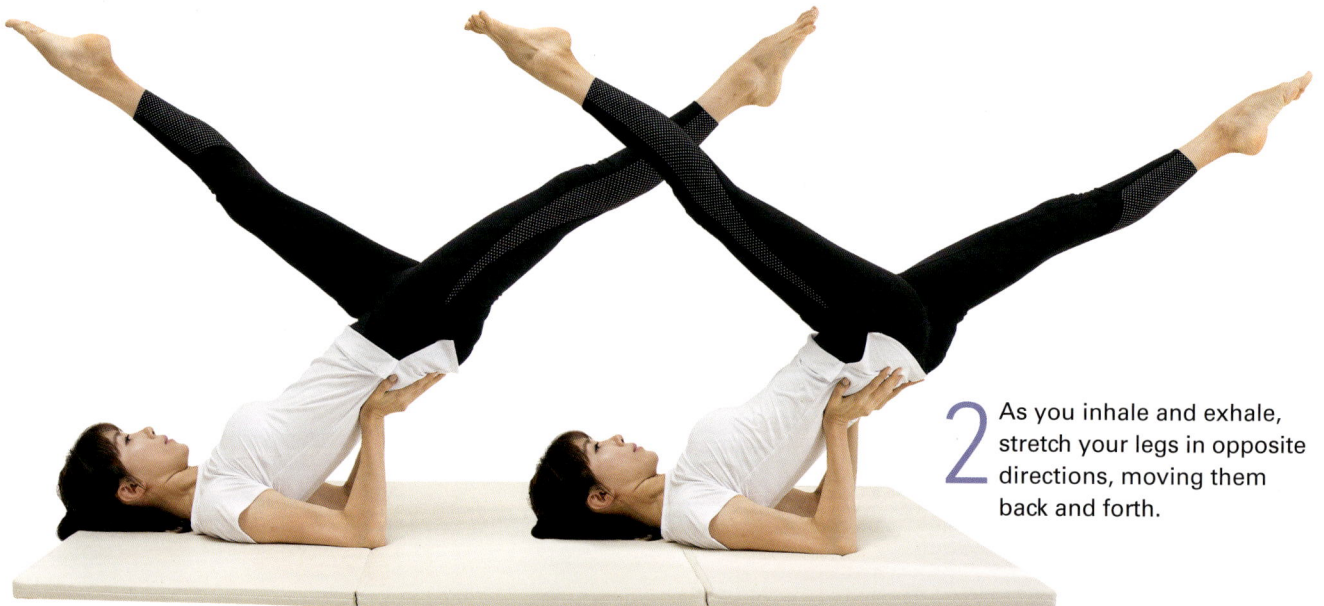

2 As you inhale and exhale, stretch your legs in opposite directions, moving them back and forth.

* Repeat five times on each leg for 10 sets.

Variation

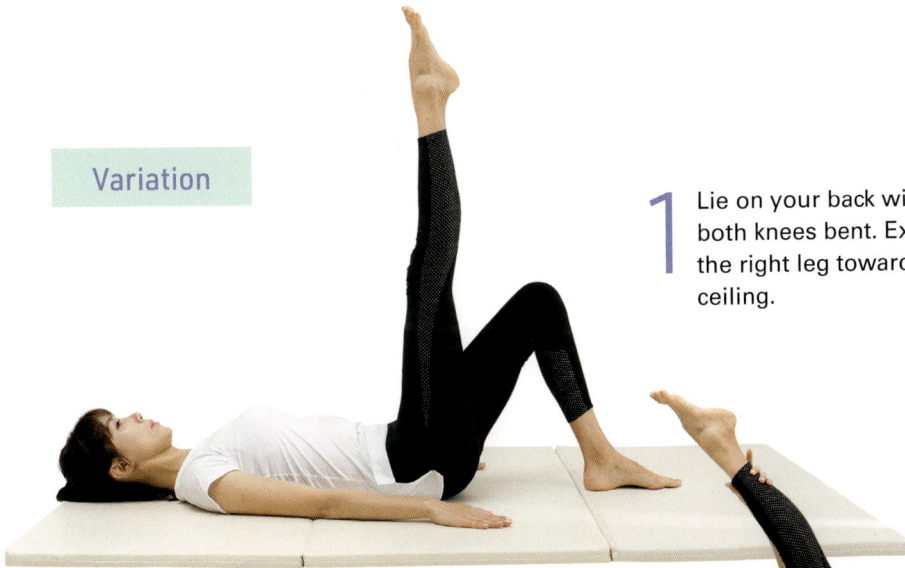

1 Lie on your back with both knees bent. Extend the right leg toward the ceiling.

2 Grab your right leg with both hands and bring it toward your chest.

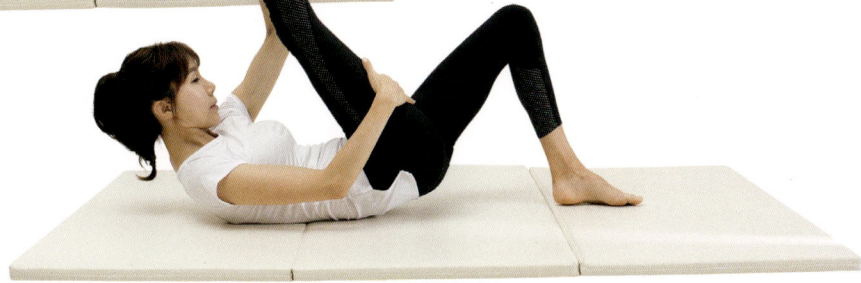

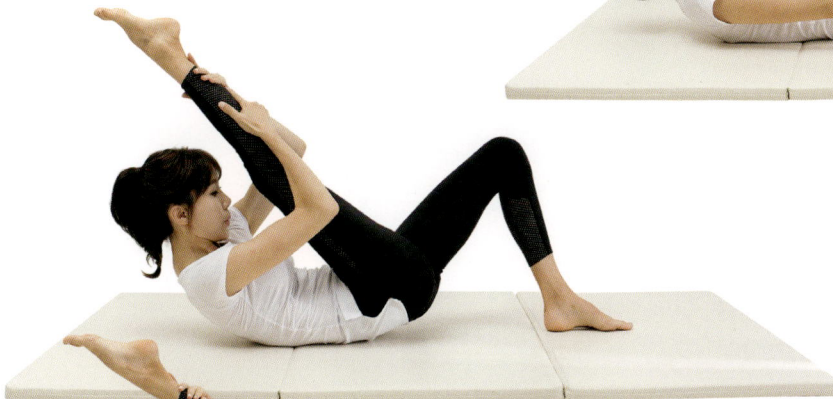

3 Tighten your abdomen and lift up your torso.

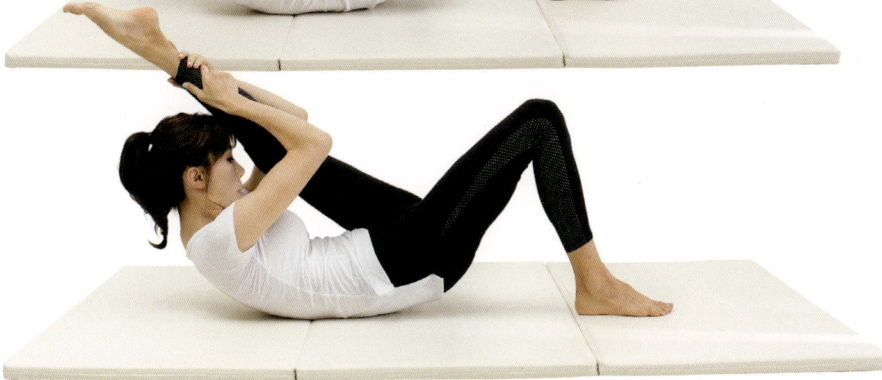

4 Alternate legs while maintaining the position.

— Tip —

The Scissors exercise has several variations. You can perform the movement with your back flat on the mat or your upper back lifted. You can mix these variations by performing movement 2 with your back flat on the floor or even try lateral scissors. Choose the option that best matches your current range of motion and strength.

Shoulder Bridge

This exercise strengthens the femoral region and helps align the erector spinae muscles and pelvis. It can also increase blood circulation, improving cardiovascular function.

1 Lie flat on your back with your knees pelvis-width apart.

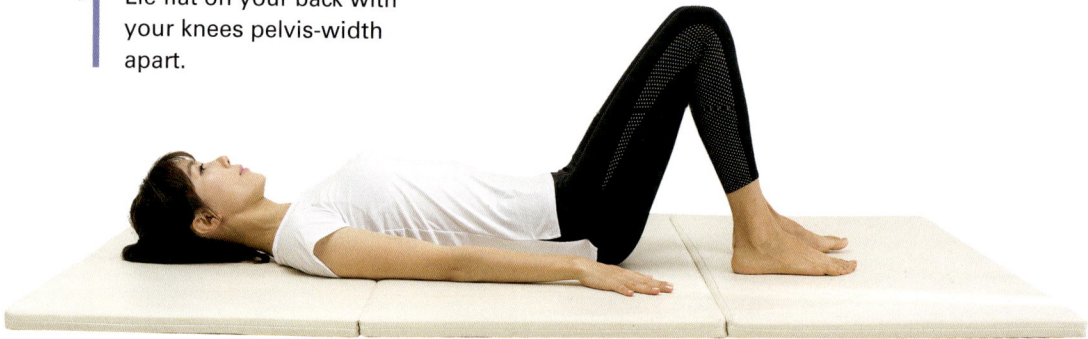

2 Lift up your pelvis as you inhale.

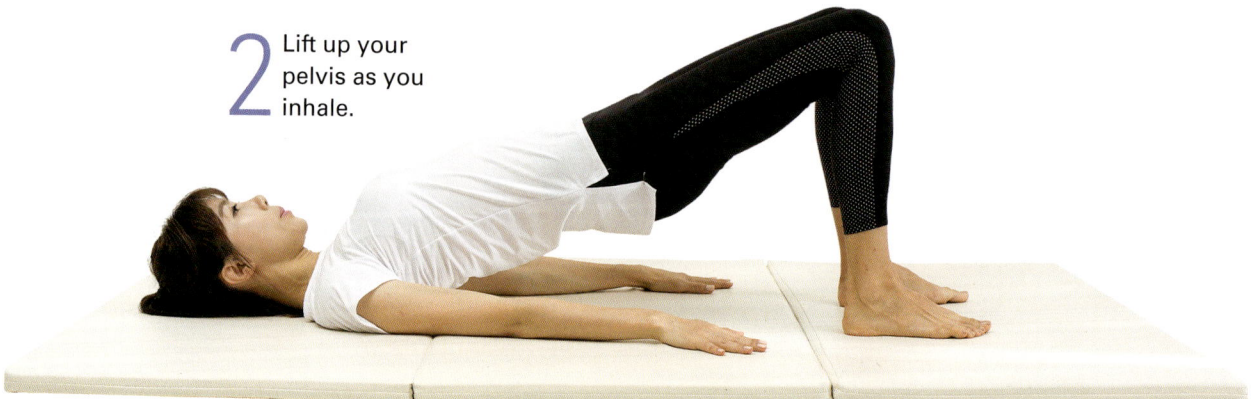

3 Support your torso with both hands.

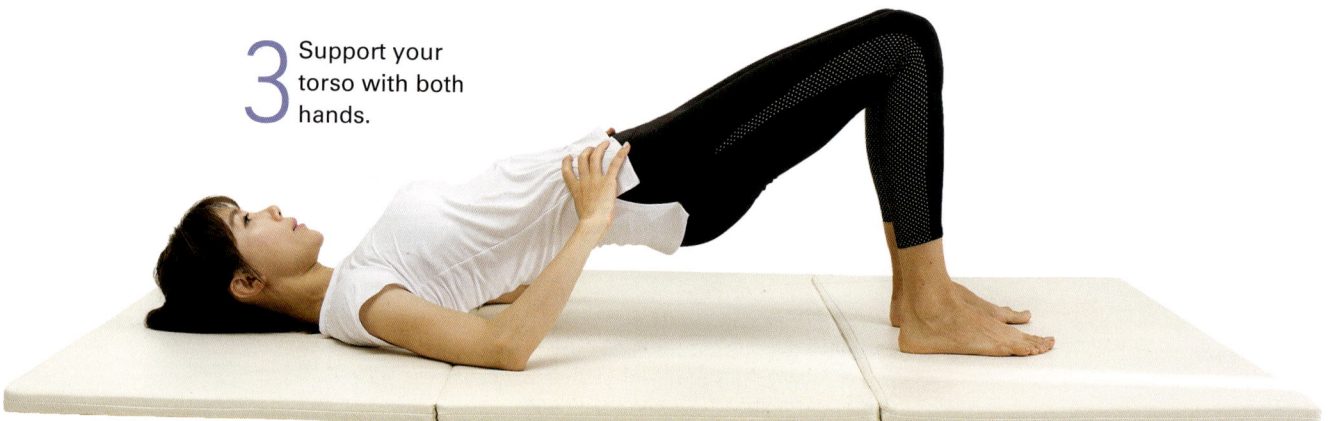

102

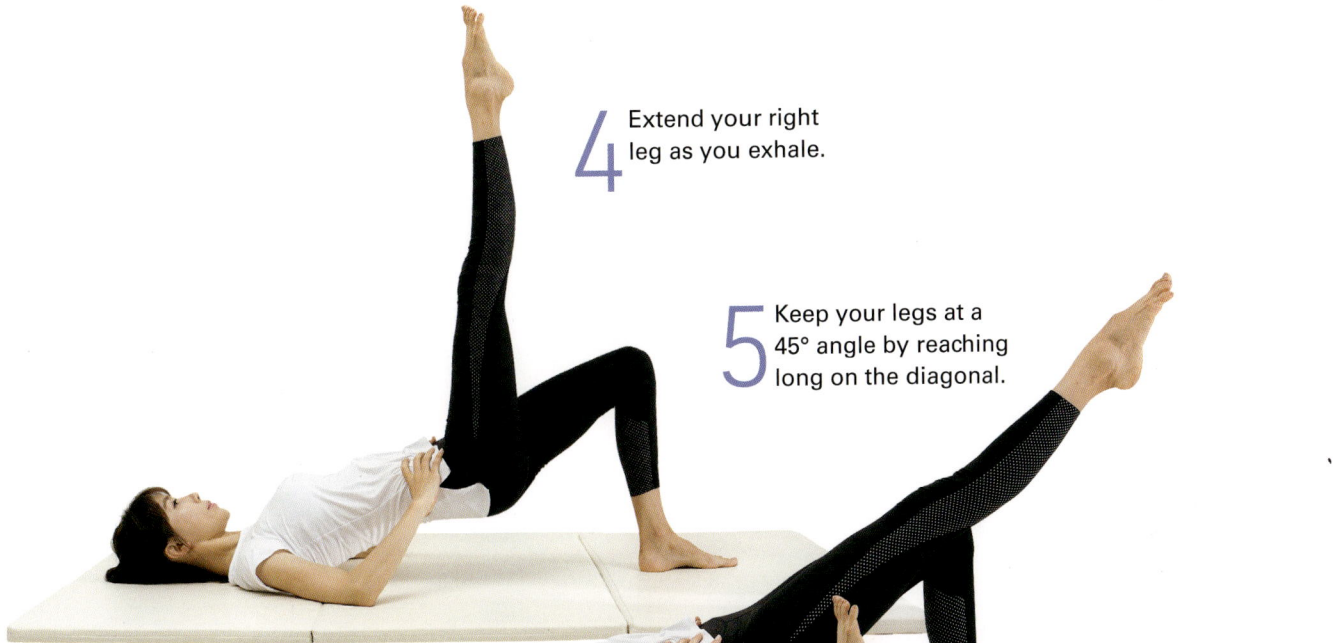

4 Extend your right leg as you exhale.

5 Keep your legs at a 45° angle by reaching long on the diagonal.

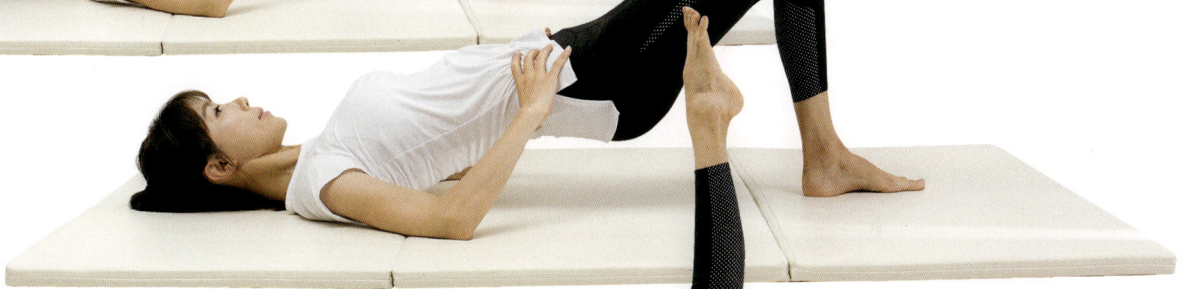

45°

6 Extend your legs up again as you inhale, and reach long on the diagonal as you exhale. Repeat several times.

* Repeat movements 4 and 5 eight times.

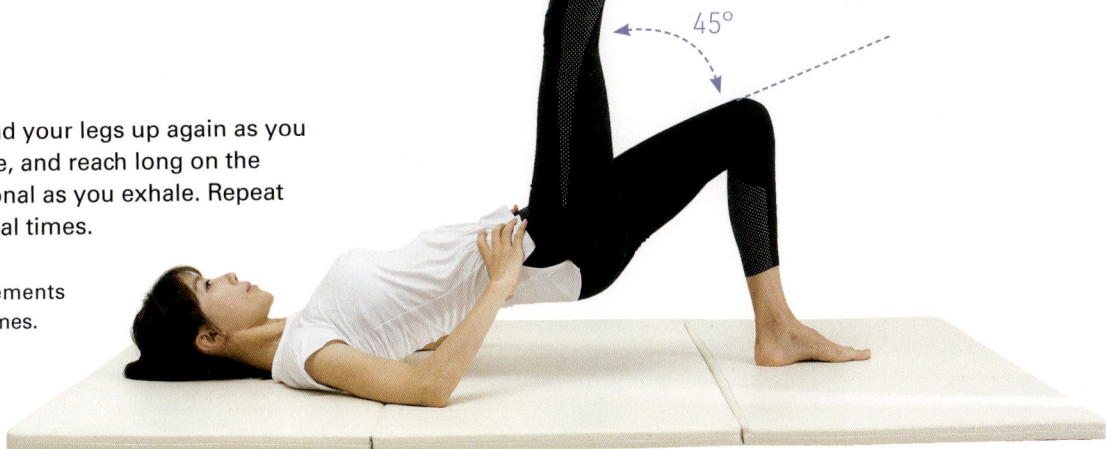

Tip

Focus on keeping your body still without collapsing. Try to maintain the same height and angle for the legs, which should be about 45° between the stretched and supporting legs. If you lack back flexibility or strength in your wrist to support the pelvis, use a prop to support your back.

103

Double-Leg Stretch

This exercise tones the abdominal area by strengthening the core muscles and enhances overall body control.

1 Lie flat on your back comfortably to begin.

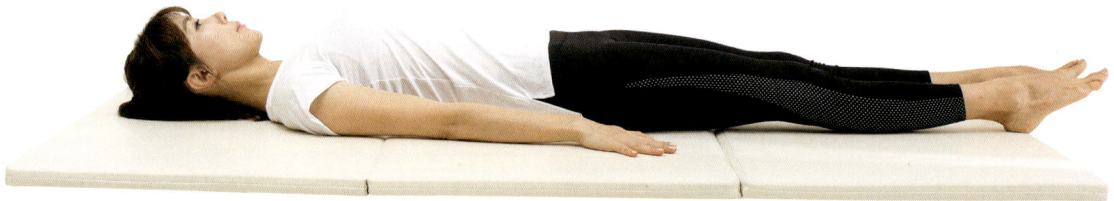

2 Bring both knees toward your chest as you inhale.

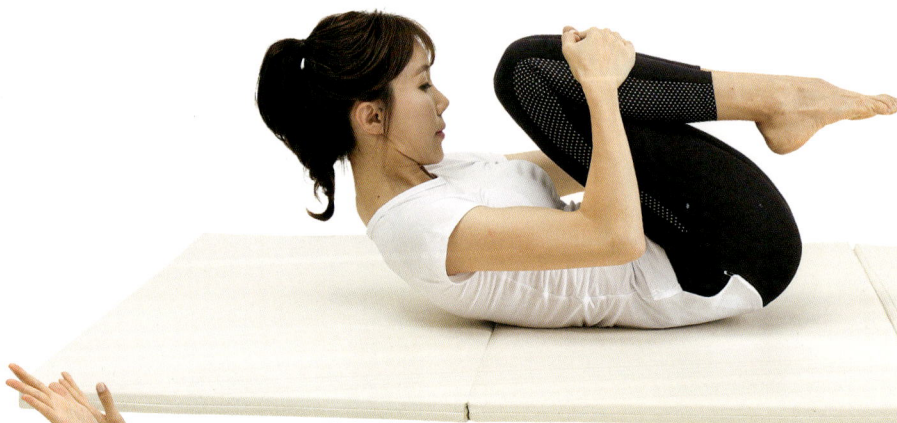

3 Extend you arms and legs as you exhale.

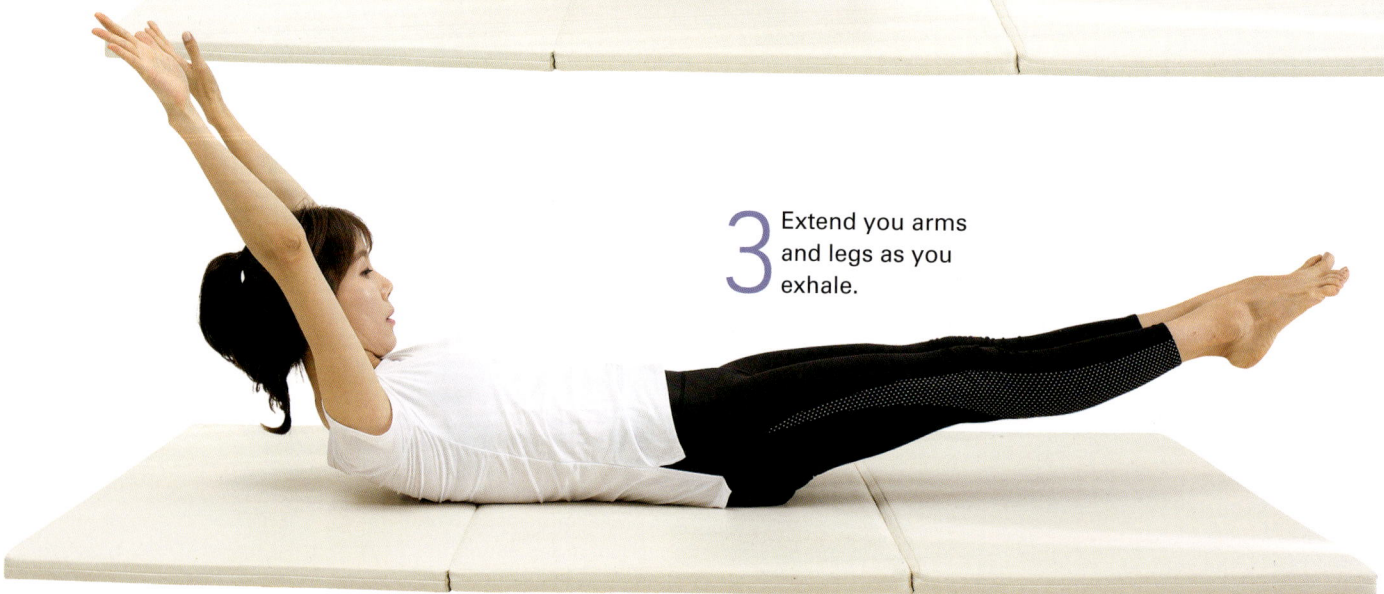

4 Inhale as you circle your arms out and around, bringing them back to your knees as you bend and hold them.

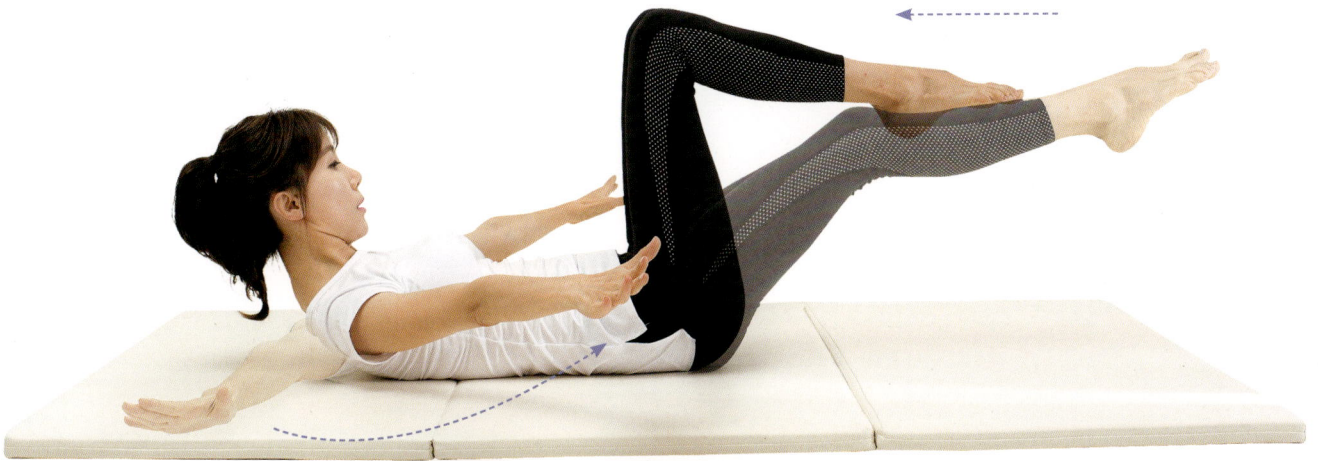

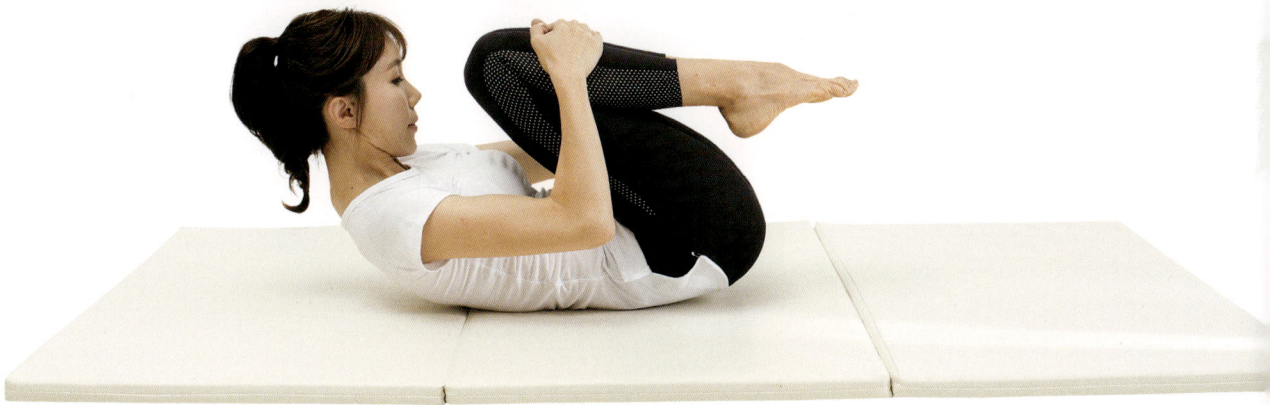

* Repeat eight times.

─Tip─

Practice the movement so you can connect each step smoothly while breathing comfortably. Repeat eight times, then return to the starting position to stretch your neck and release any tension.

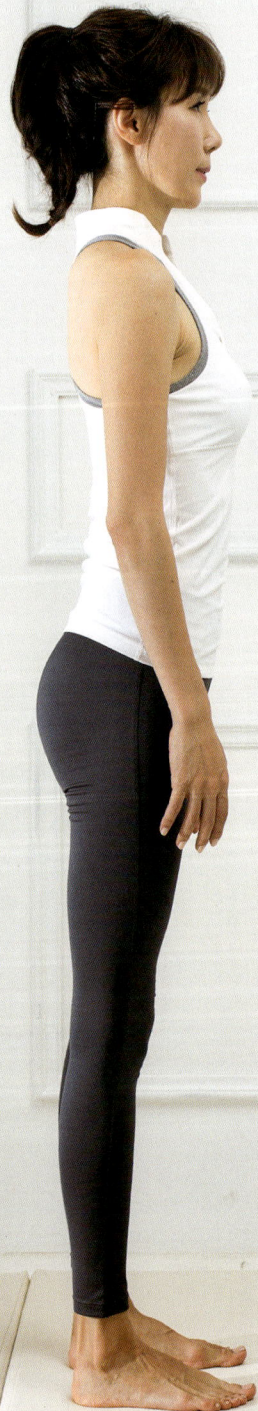

Neutral Posture

Many exercises begin and end with the standing position. This posture helps you restore balance and calm your breathing. Stand comfortably, feeling the effects of gravity and becoming aware of your body.

Focus on engaging your core as you breathe, and maintain the natural curve of your spine to avoid overstraining your back.

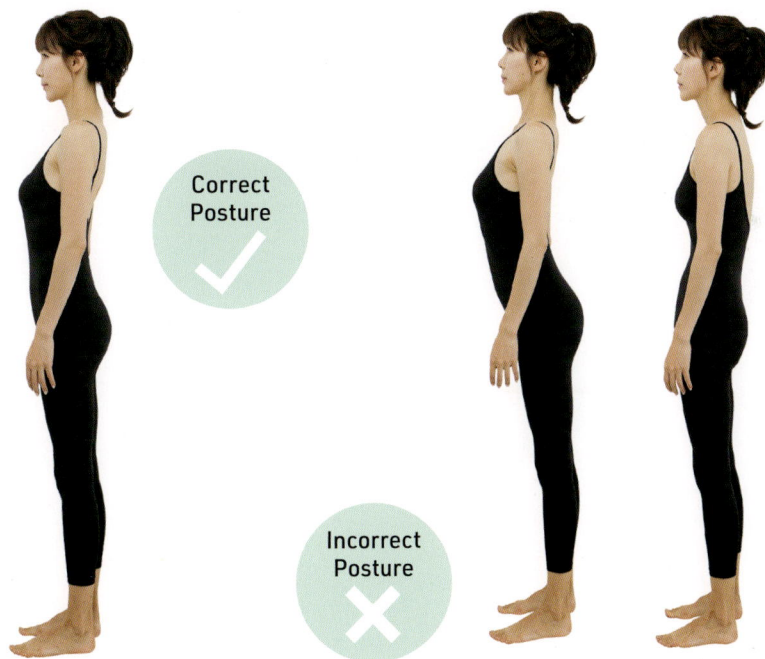

Correct
Posture

Incorrect
Posture

Standing Roll-Down

This exercise can help you build a supple spine and increase lower-body flexibility. It can also help relieve tension and reduce headaches.

1 Stand straight with your legs pelvis-width apart and inhale to begin.

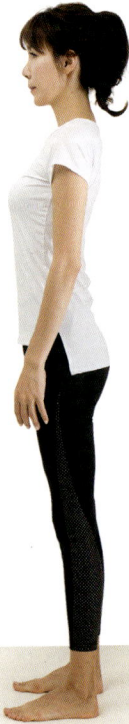

2 Bend your head down as you exhale.

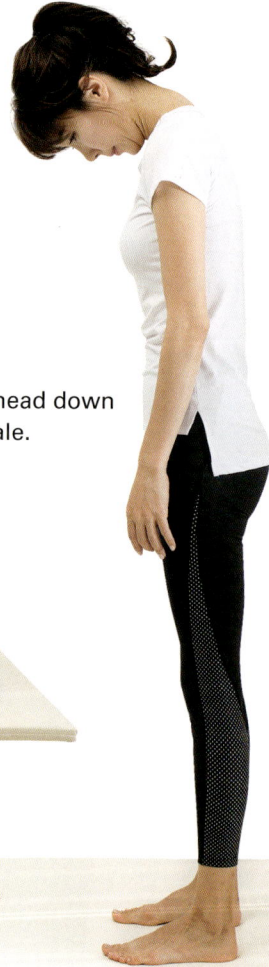

3 Slowly lower your torso, feeling each vertebra, one at a time, from the top of your neck to the base of your spine.

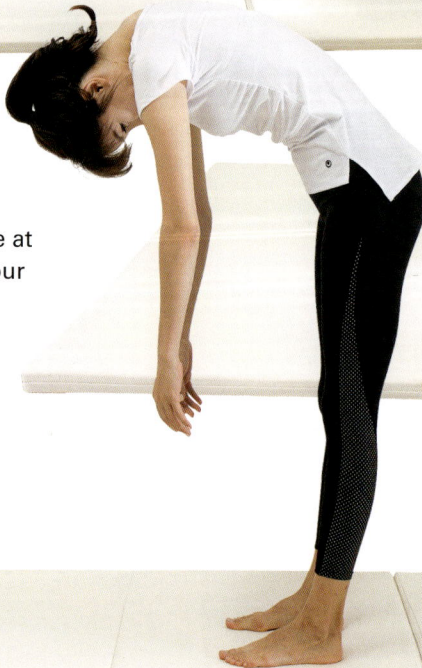

4 Extend your legs by moving the center of gravity more to the front without touching your hands to the ground.

5 Turn your head to the left and right. Let your arms circle loosely near the floor. Slowly lift your torso, feeling each vertebra.

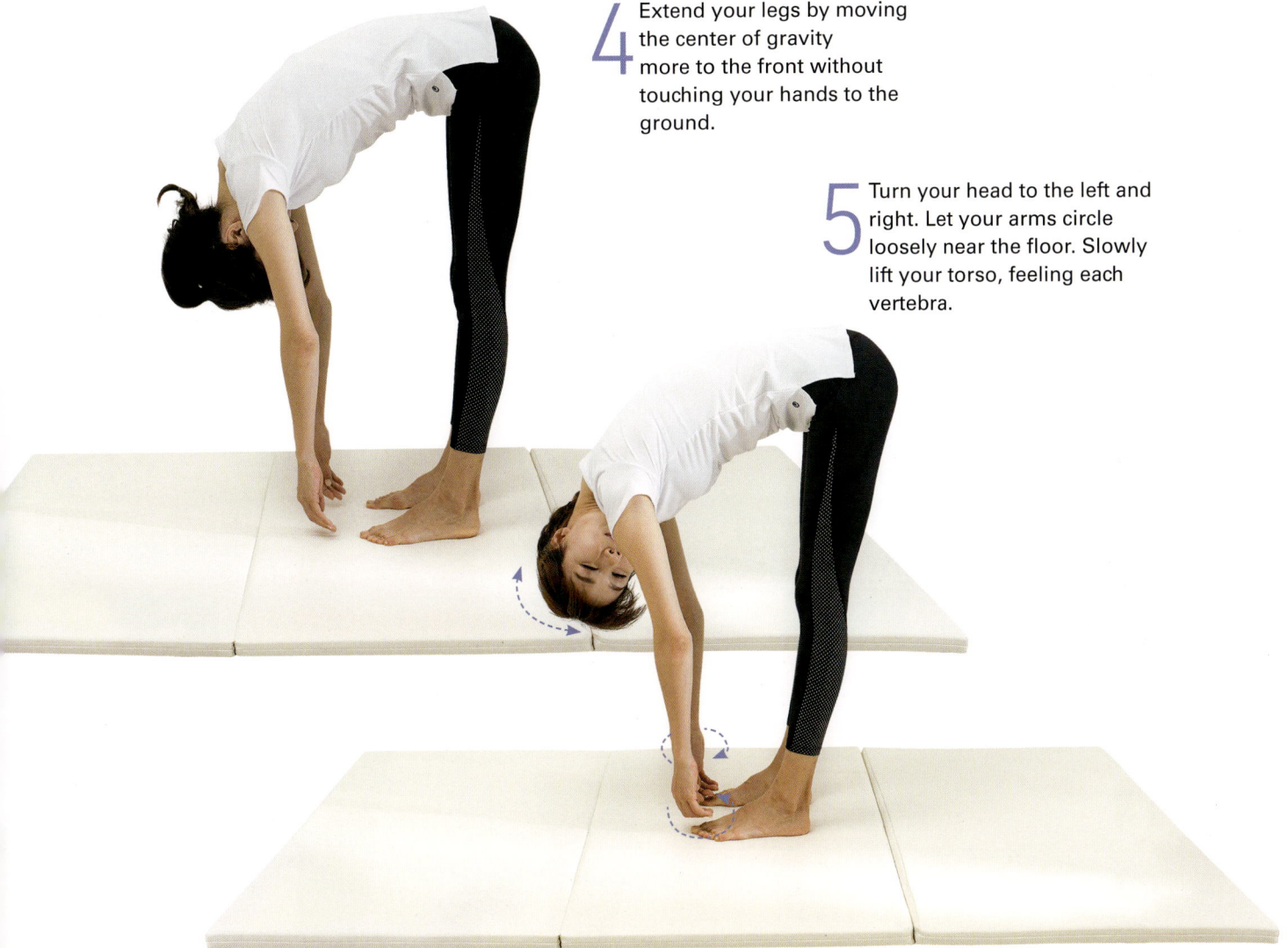

*Repeat movements 1 to 5 two times.

Tip

If you have spinal concerns or experience difficulty, progress slowly by starting with your hands on your legs. You might find it difficult to straighten your knees if you lack leg flexibility, but maintaining straight legs is essential for proper form. Work within your current range of flexibility.

Pilates Breathing

This exercise helps you finish your workout with mindful breathing. Taking deep breaths will calm the heart rate, regulate body temperature, and release any remaining tension.

1 Stand straight with your legs pelvis-width apart and put your hands together to begin.

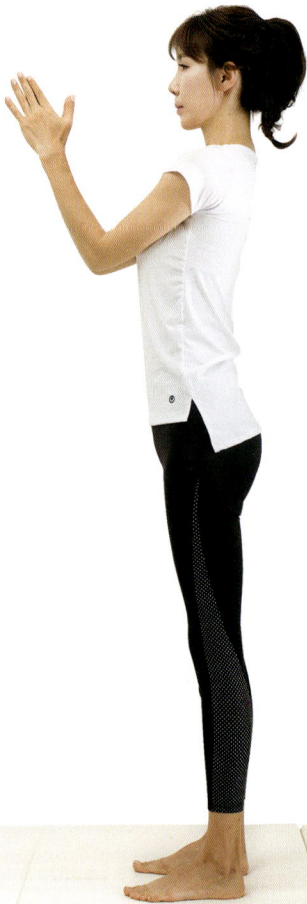

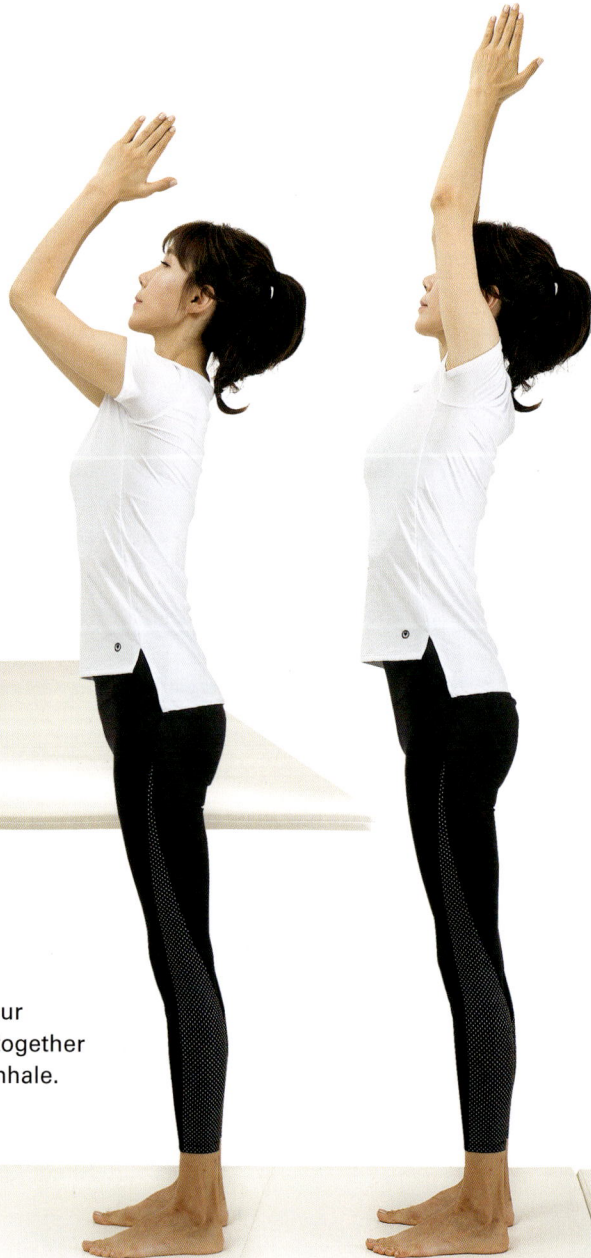

2 Raise your elbows together as you inhale.

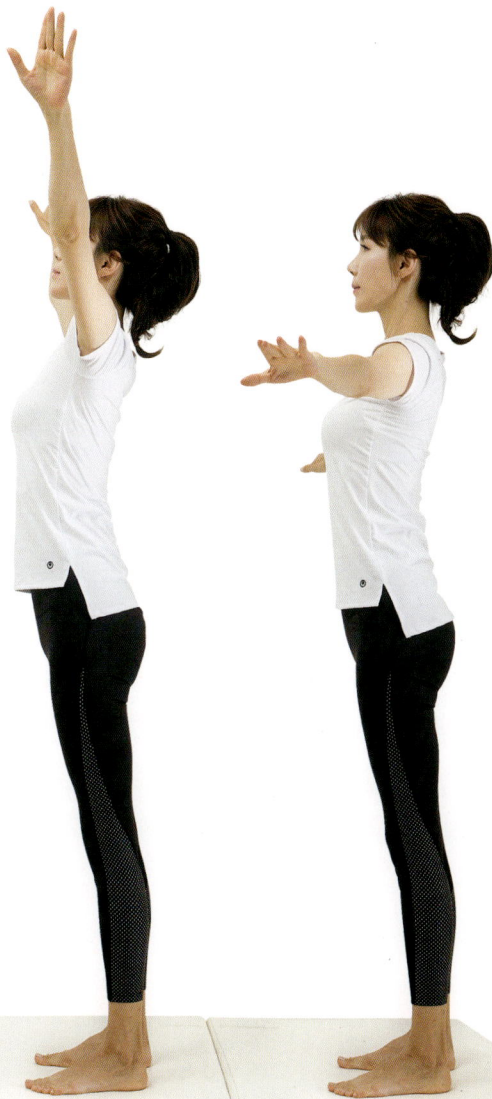

3 Draw a big circle with both arms over your head as you exhale.

4 Slowly bring your arms down.

* Keep both arms within your sight.

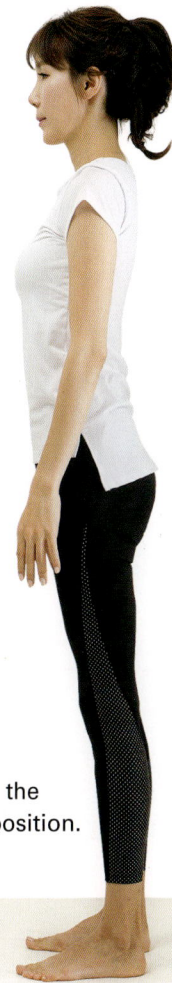

5 Return to the starting position.

* Repeat movements 1 to 5 five times.

Tip

Make sure you don't open your chest wide or bend backward as you raise your elbows.

Pilates with Props

Pilates often utilizes props for maximum results. Props can help by adding resistance, increasing stability, and aiding alignment. Instead of using the specialized tools from a studio, you can achieve great results at home by using simple tools such as a foam roller, gym ball, Pilates ring, or resistance band for various movements easily adapted to different fitness levels.

Foam Roller

Neck Stretching	This exercise can release tension around the neck and shoulders by gently stretching surrounding muscles.

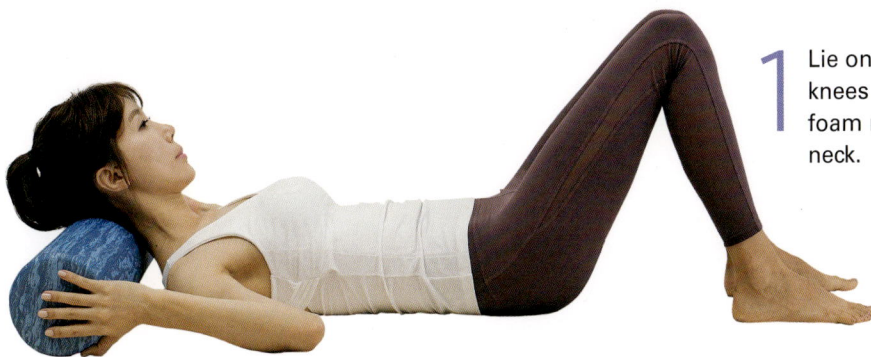

1 Lie on your back with your knees bent and place the foam roller behind your neck.

2 Pull your chin toward your chest, elongating the back of your neck. Turn your head left and right to relieve tightness.

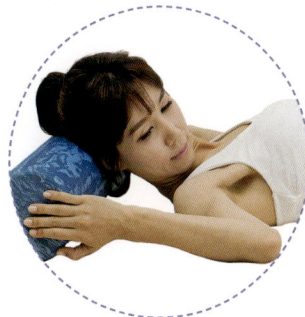

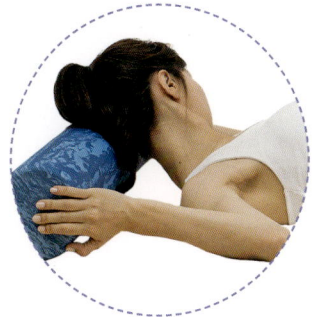

Shoulder Stretching

This exercise can help correct rounded shoulders and prevent frozen shoulder.

1 Place a foam roller on the floor and carefully lie along it, supported from head to tailbone.

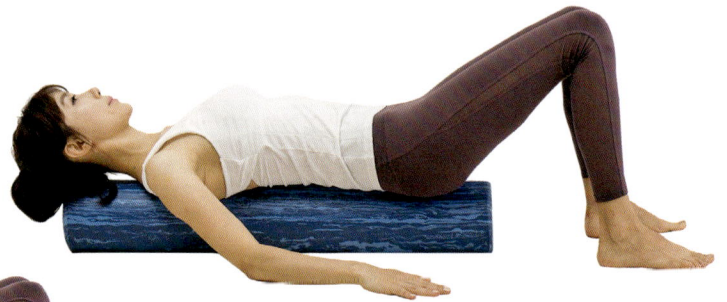

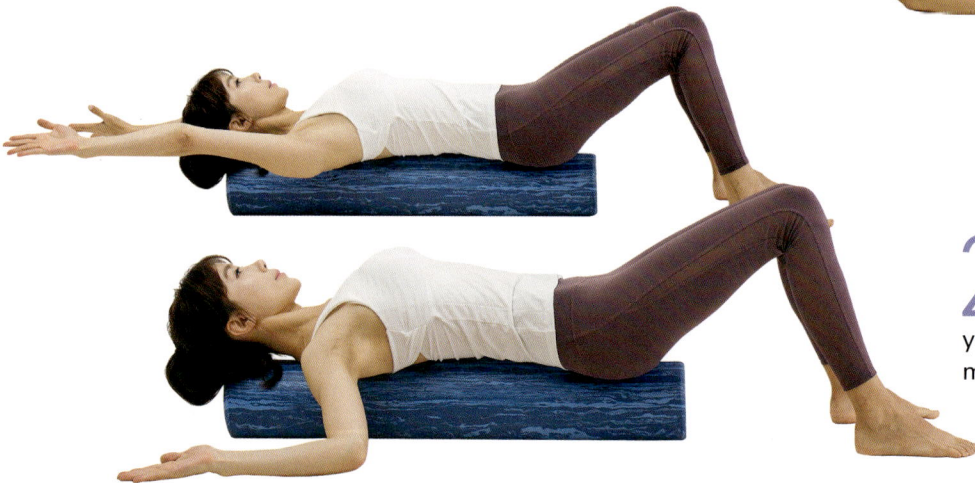

2 Raise your arms overhead, then lower the arms as you rotate your shoulders and relax the muscles.

Upper Body Stretching

This exercise helps correct spinal curvature and aids in digestion by stimulating the solar plexus area.

1 Lie on your back with both knees bent. Place foam roller behind your back to begin.

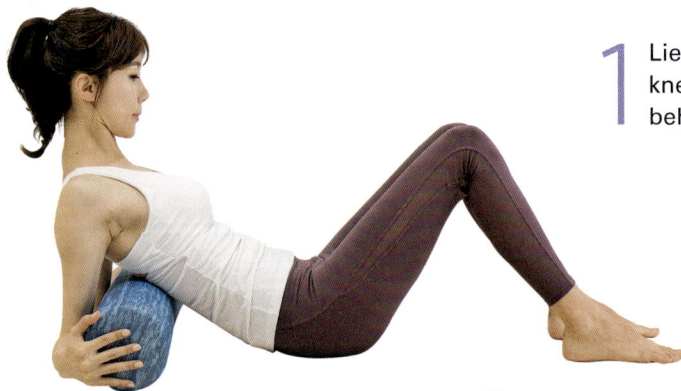

2 With both hands supporting your head, lean your torso back. Lift up your torso by rounding your spine.

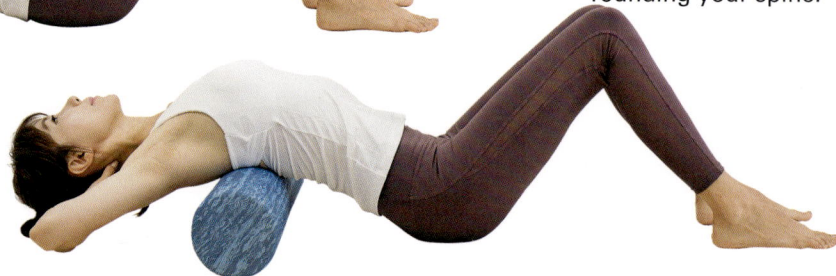

114

Lower Body Stretching

This exercise helps relax the legs and reduce swelling by gently massaging the lower body muscles.

1 Balance on your elbows and tighten the sphincter muscle to keep your legs straight.

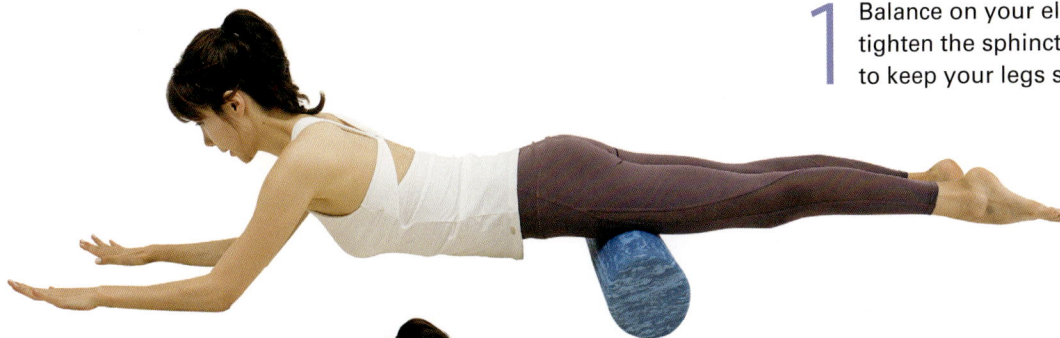

2 Move back and forth, using your body weight to massage the front of your thighs.

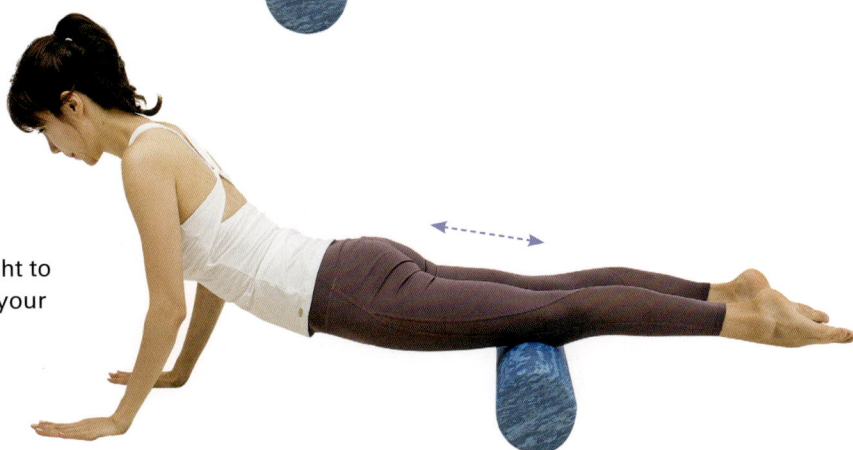

3 Place the foam roller under your legs and massage the back of your thighs as in the previous movement.

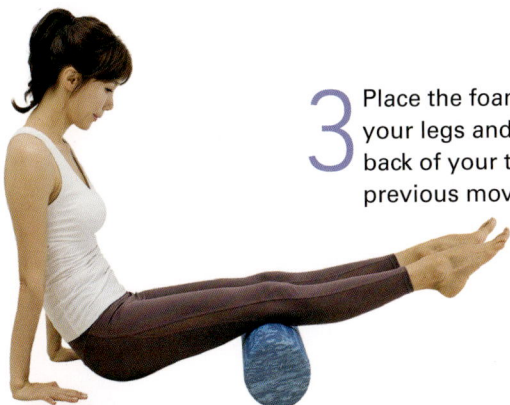

4 Massage your upper thighs as in the previous movement. Keep your arms bent in a comfortable position.

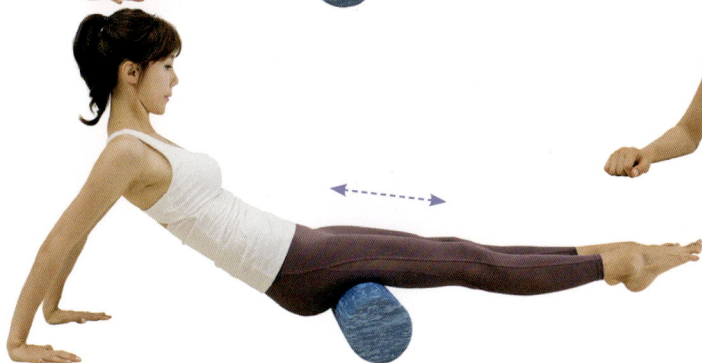

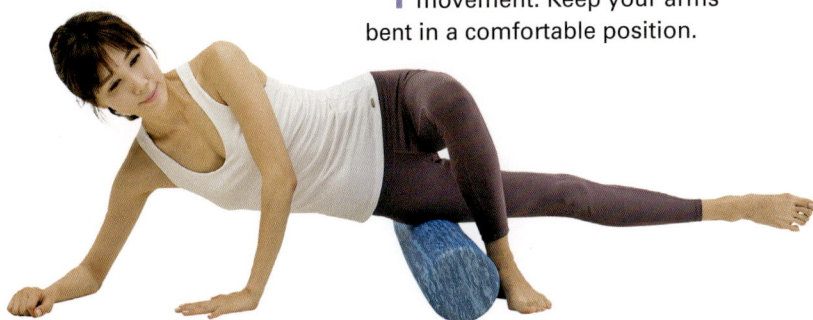

Back of the Body Stretching

This exercise helps relax the backside of the body—back, waist, and legs. It also increases flexibility.

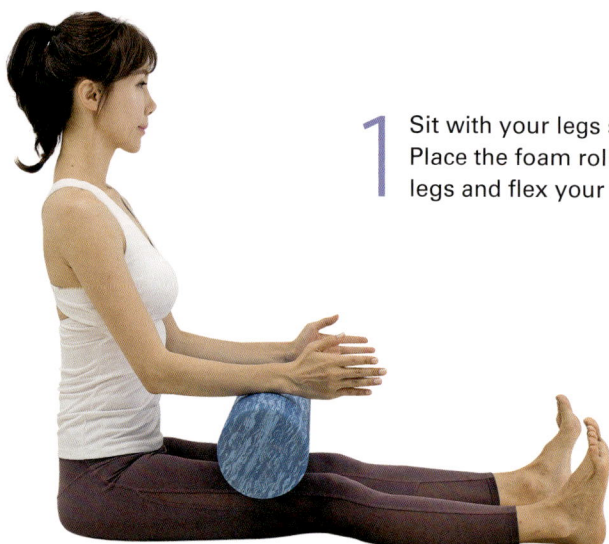

1 Sit with your legs stretched. Place the foam roller on your legs and flex your feet to begin.

2 Roll the foam roller forward as you inhale and lower your torso slowly while elongating your spine.

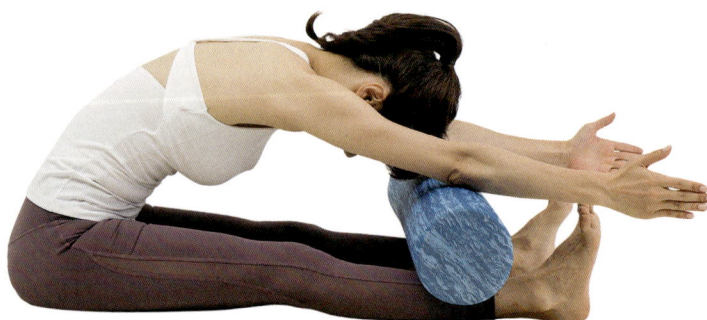

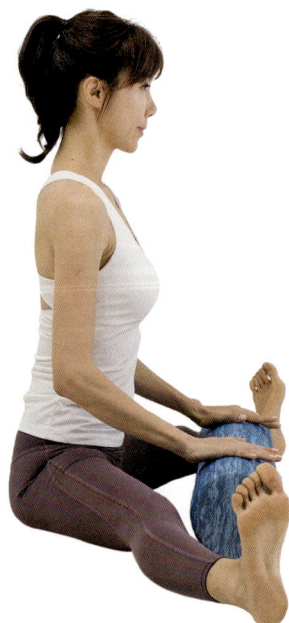

3 Practice the exercise with your legs wide apart. Roll the foam roller forward and lower your torso as you elongate your spine.

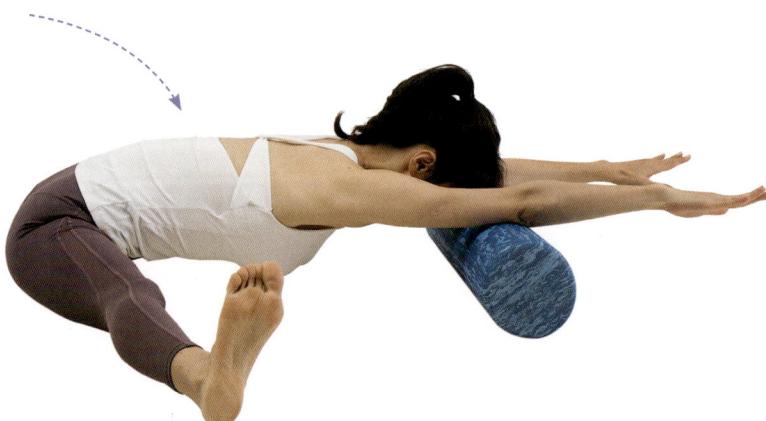

Curl Up

This is one of the best exercises to tone the stomach area and strengthen the upper abdominal muscles.

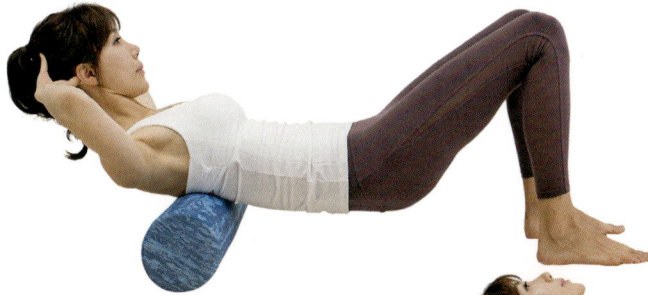

1 Lie on your back and place the foam roller under your upper back. Place both hands next to your ears.

2 Lean your body back as you inhale. Stop before you touch the ground.

3 Curl up your torso as you exhale.

* Lean back as you inhale and lift up as you exhale. Repeat several times.

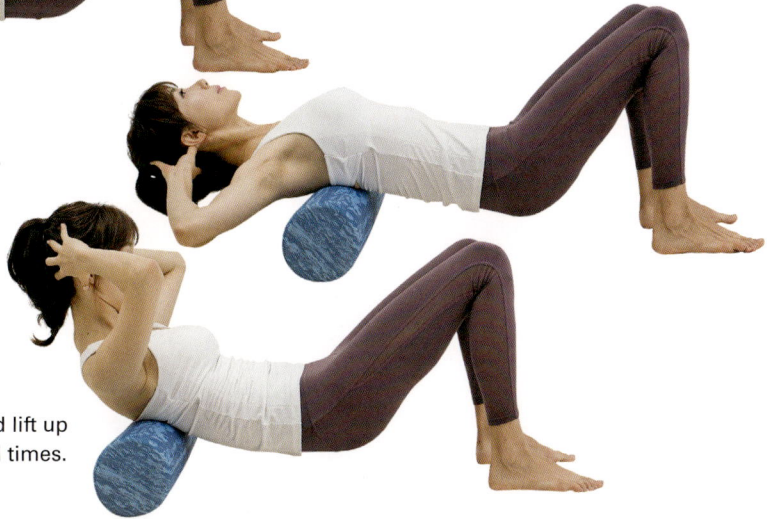

Leg Raise

This is another great exercise to tone the stomach area and strengthen the lower abdominal muscles.

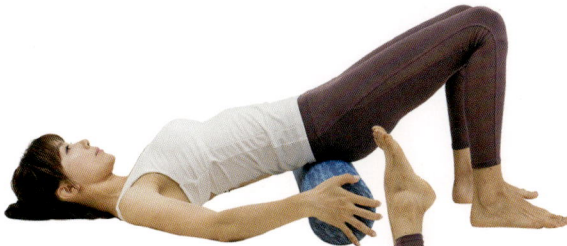

1 Lie with your knees bent and place the foam roller behind your pelvis.

2 Inhale and raise your legs until they are perpendicular to the floor.

3 Exhale and lower your legs to a 45° angle from the floor.

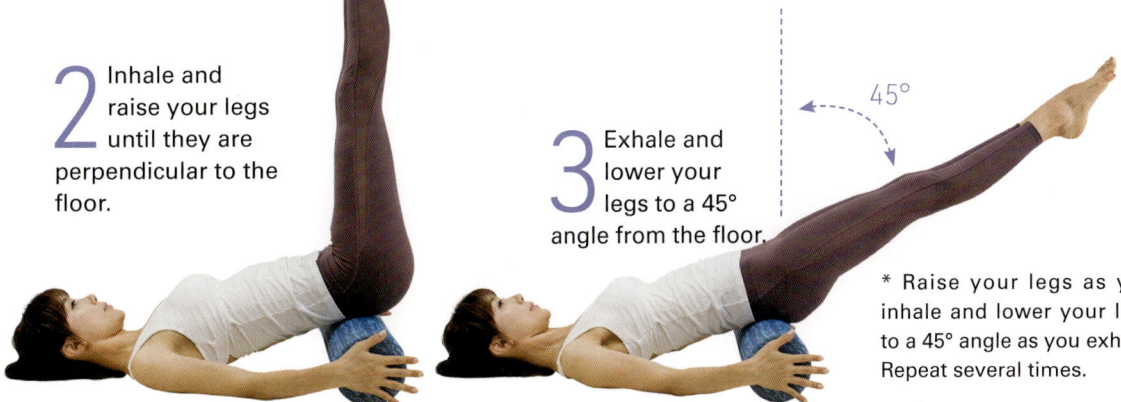

45°

* Raise your legs as you inhale and lower your legs to a 45° angle as you exhale. Repeat several times.

Single-Leg Stretch This exercise can improve core strength and flexibility and also increase blood circulation in the lower body.

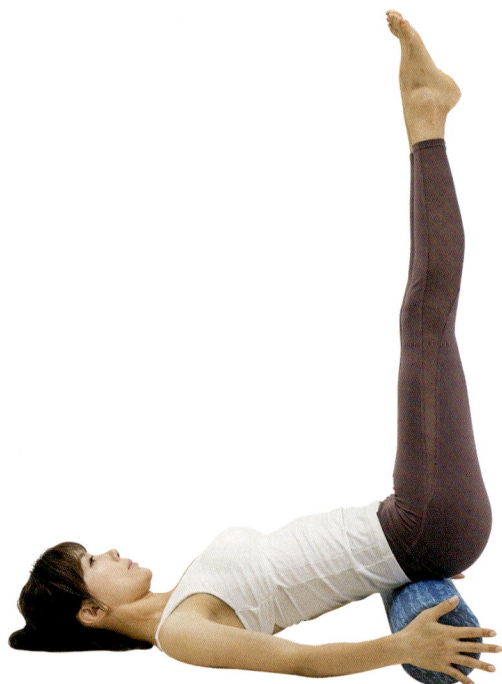

1 Place the foam roller behind your pelvis. Spread your legs as wide as you can. Repeat the movement in a scissor-like motion.

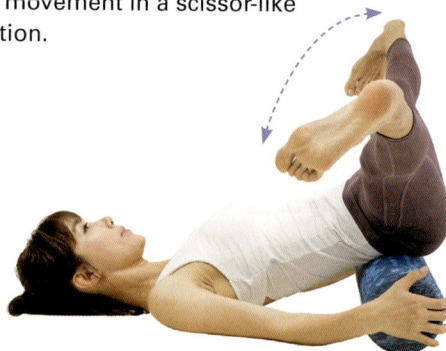

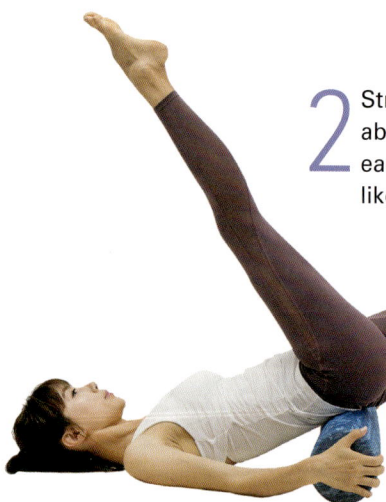

2 Strengthen your abdomen by alternating each leg back and forth like a scissor.

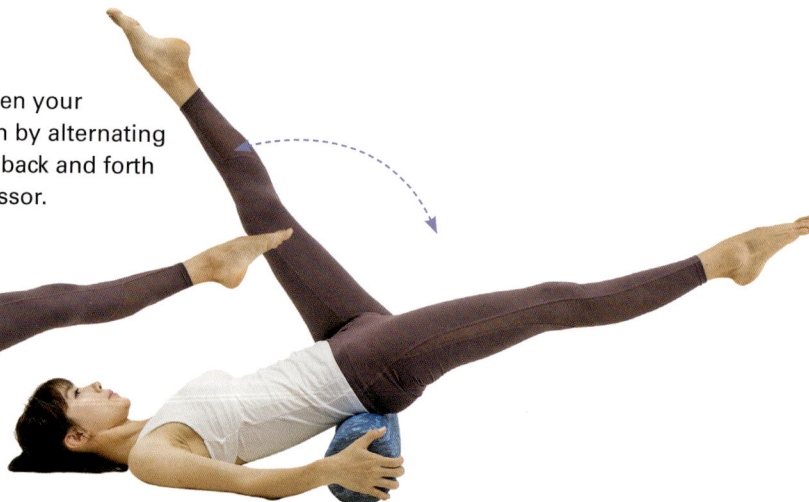

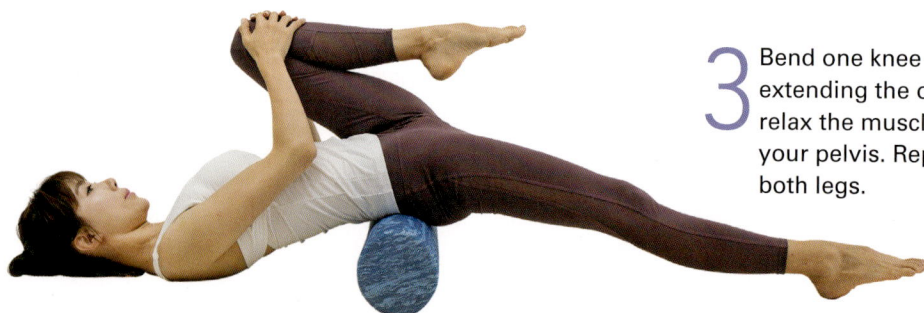

3 Bend one knee while extending the other to relax the muscles around your pelvis. Repeat on both legs.

The Swan	This exercise can tone shoulders, back, and hips by strengthening the erector spinae muscles.

1 Lie on your belly and place the foam roller under your forearms to begin.

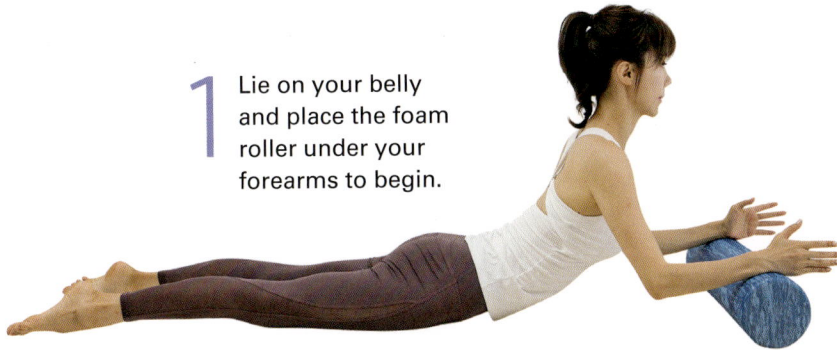

2 Roll the foam roller forward as you exhale. Lower your torso and raise your legs up. Keep your hips tight.

* Roll the foam roller back and forth with your body.

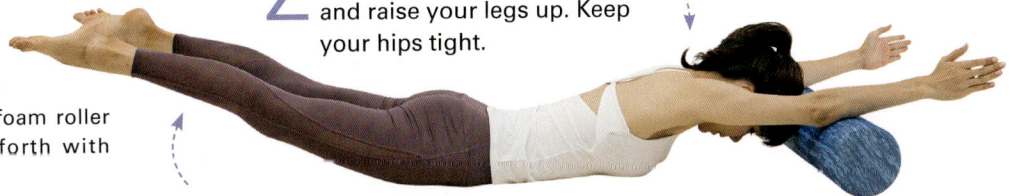

Squat	This exercise can improve the lower body muscles and tone the legs and hips.

1 Lean on a wall and place the foam roller behind your pelvis.

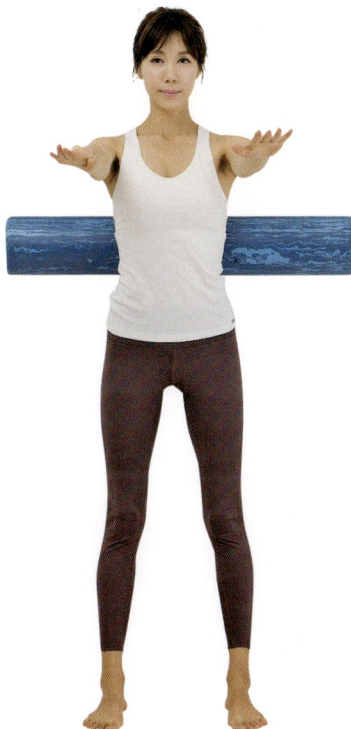

2 Exhale and bend your knees to 90°. Inhale and stand up while tightening your thighs and hips.

* To increase the challenge, you can also exercise with your heels up.

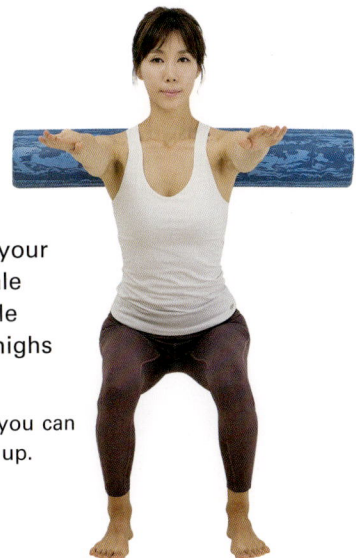

Pilates Ring

This exercise can tone the upper body, aid digestion, and release stress.

1 Stand with your feet shoulder-width apart. Hold the ring with both hands to begin.

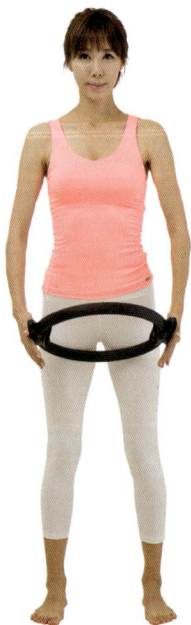

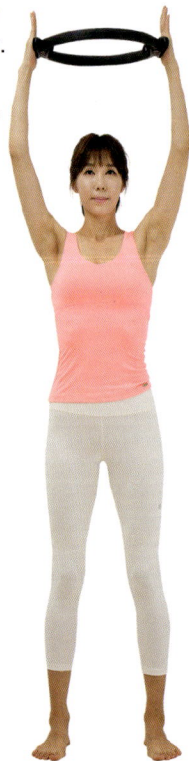

2 Raise your arms as you inhale.

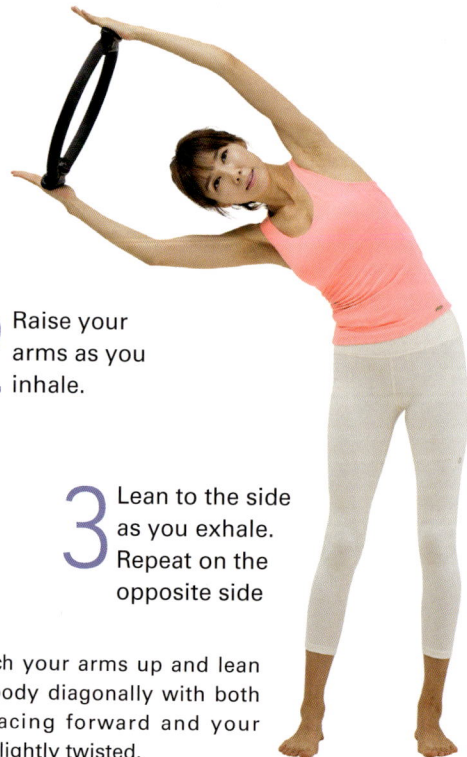

3 Lean to the side as you exhale. Repeat on the opposite side

* Reach your arms up and lean your body diagonally with both legs facing forward and your body slightly twisted.

Full-Body Stretching

This exercise helps relieve overall body tension while increasing flexibility in the shoulders, chest, back, and legs.

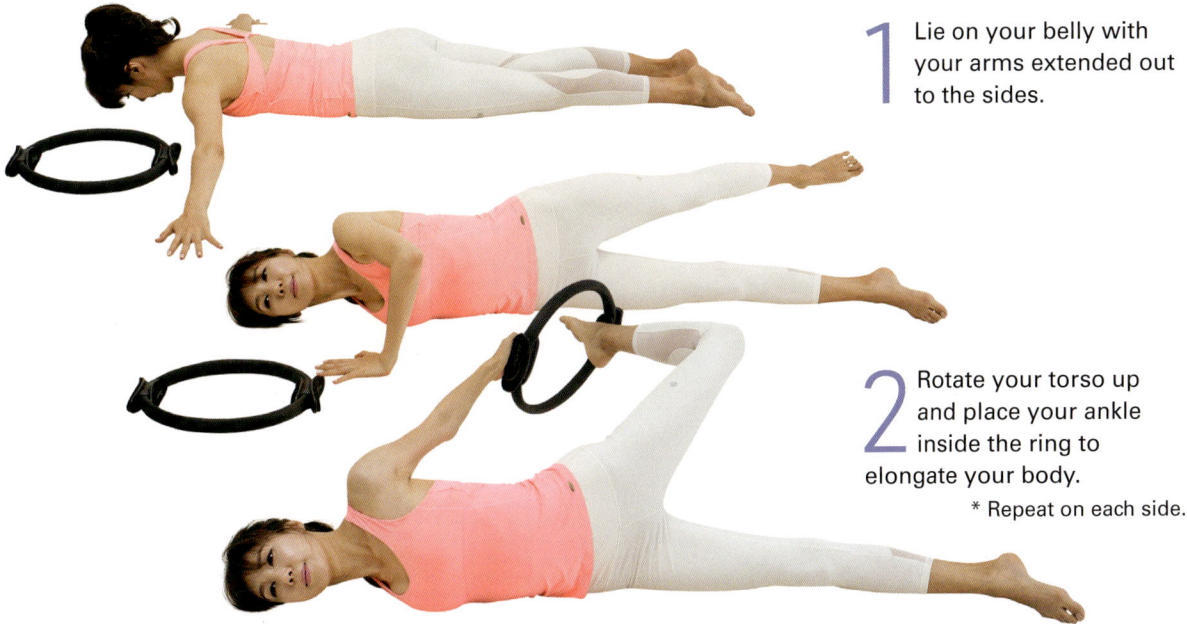

1 Lie on your belly with your arms extended out to the sides.

2 Rotate your torso up and place your ankle inside the ring to elongate your body.

* Repeat on each side.

Calf Stretching

This exercise stimulates the calf muscles, often referred to as the "second heart," and boosts overall circulation.

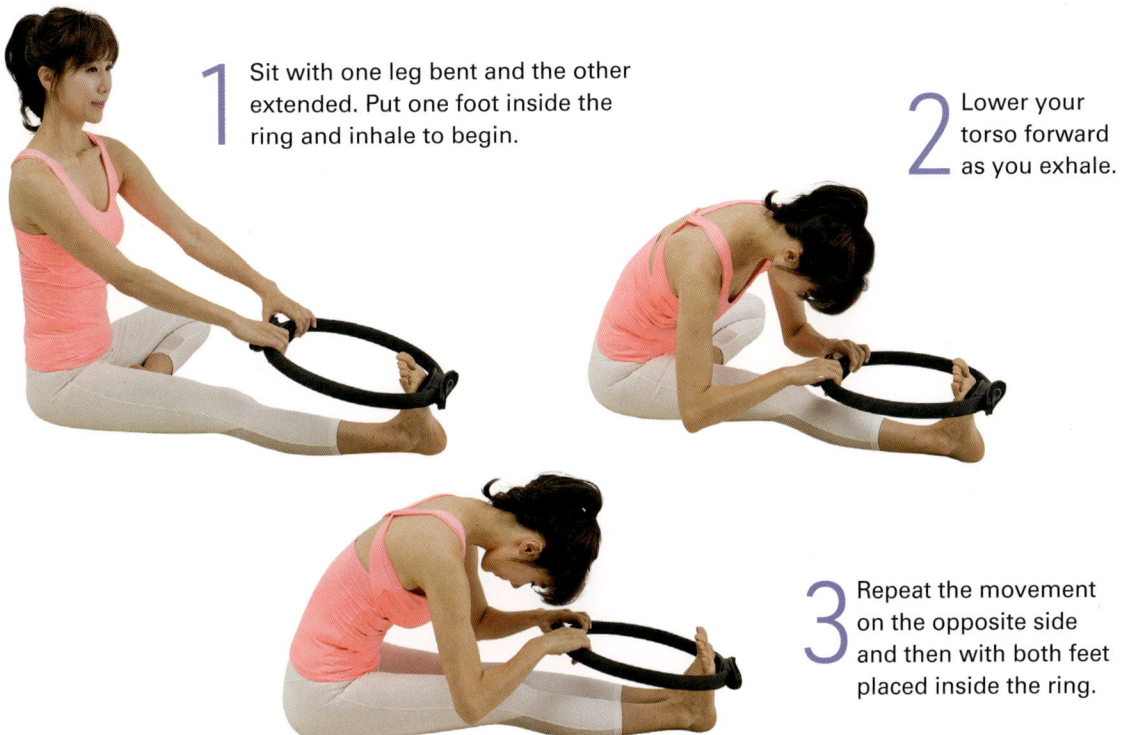

1 Sit with one leg bent and the other extended. Put one foot inside the ring and inhale to begin.

2 Lower your torso forward as you exhale.

3 Repeat the movement on the opposite side and then with both feet placed inside the ring.

Thigh Stretching

This exercise can tone the lower body while reducing nerve pain in the back and legs by relieving tension along the nerve pathways.

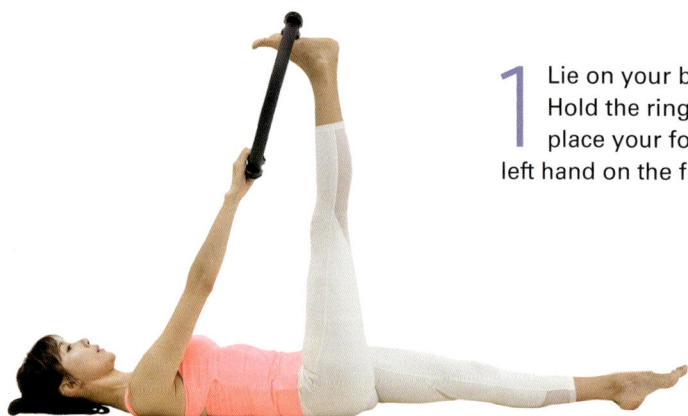

1 Lie on your back and raise your right leg. Hold the ring with your right hand and place your foot inside the ring. Rest your left hand on the floor. Inhale to begin.

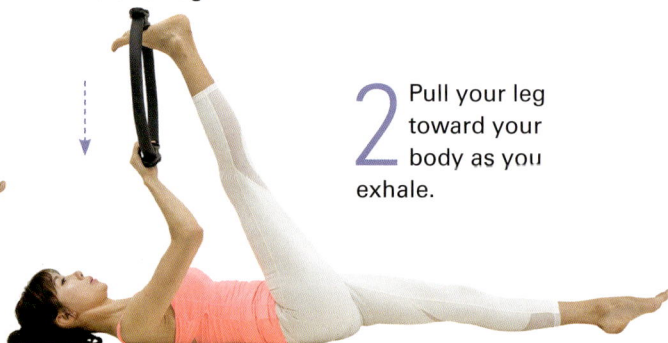

2 Pull your leg toward your body as you exhale.

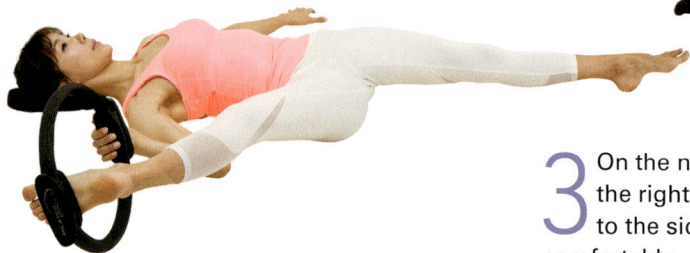

3 On the next exhale, guide the right leg outward to the side as far as comfortable.

* Repeat on both legs.

Single Leg Roll-Up

This exercise helps lengthen your spine, improving flexibility and mobility in the back and strengthening the abdominal muscles.

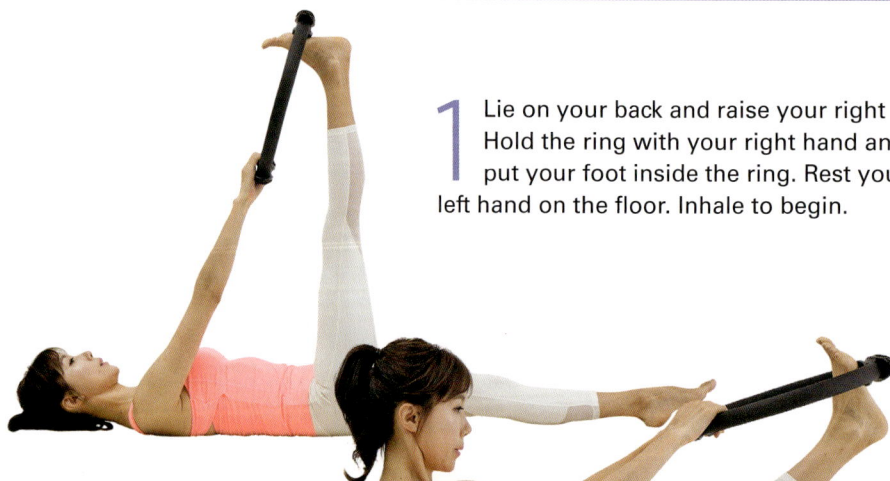

1 Lie on your back and raise your right leg. Hold the ring with your right hand and put your foot inside the ring. Rest your left hand on the floor. Inhale to begin.

2 Curl up your torso as you exhale, engaging the abdominal muscle.

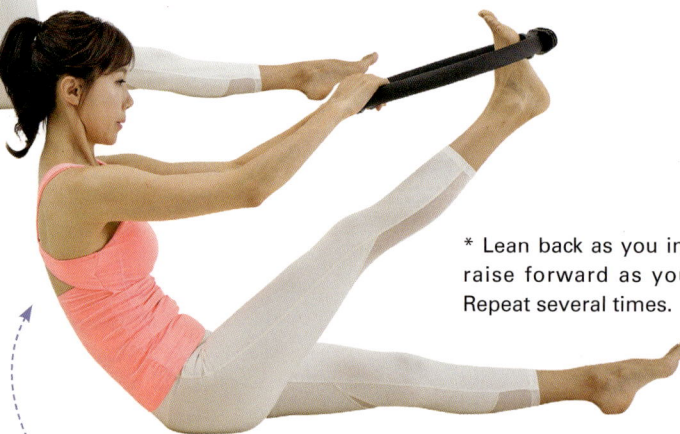

* Lean back as you inhale, and raise forward as you exhale. Repeat several times.

| This exercise can strengthen the chest muscles and tone the arms and shoulders.

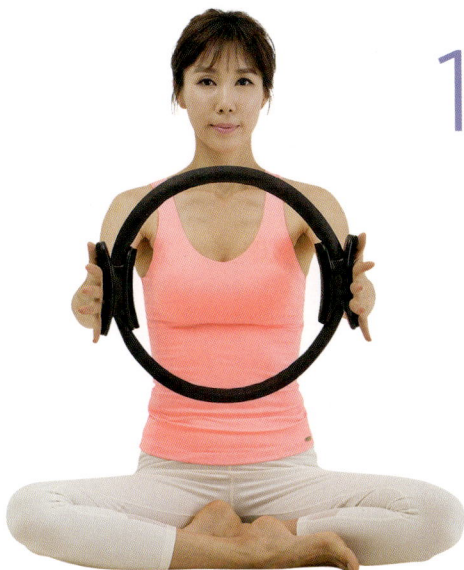

1 Sit cross-legged and stretch both arms forward while holding the ring. Keep your elbows slightly bent and relaxed.

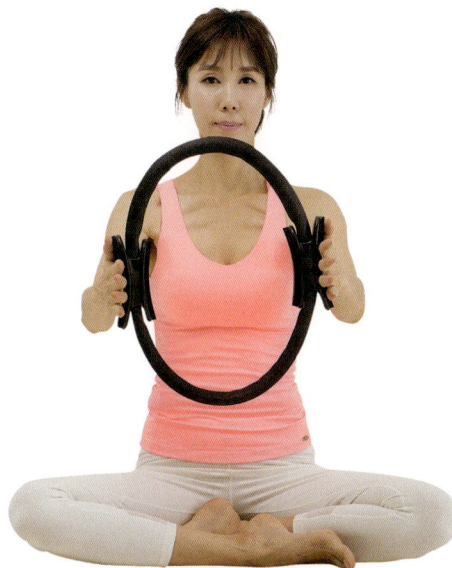

2 Slowly press the ring with both arms as you exhale, engaging the chest muscles.

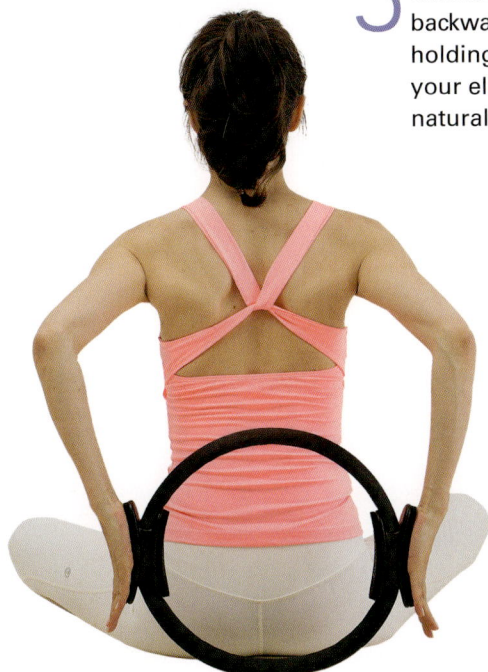

3 Sit cross-legged and extend both arms backward while holding the ring. Allow your elbows to bend naturally.

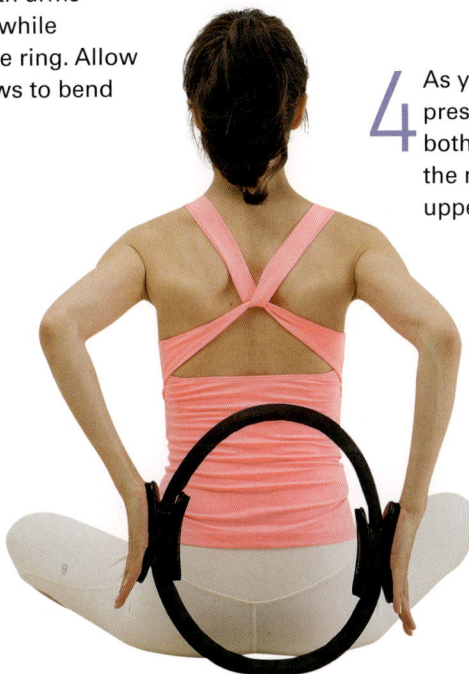

4 As you exhale, slowly press the ring using both arms, engaging the muscles of your upper back.

This exercise can tone the hips and thighs by strengthening the inner thigh muscles.

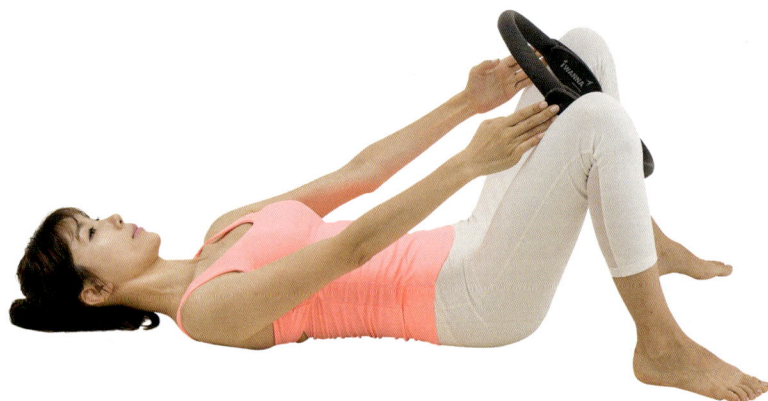

1 Lie on your back with both knees bent. Place the ring between your knees. Inhale to begin.

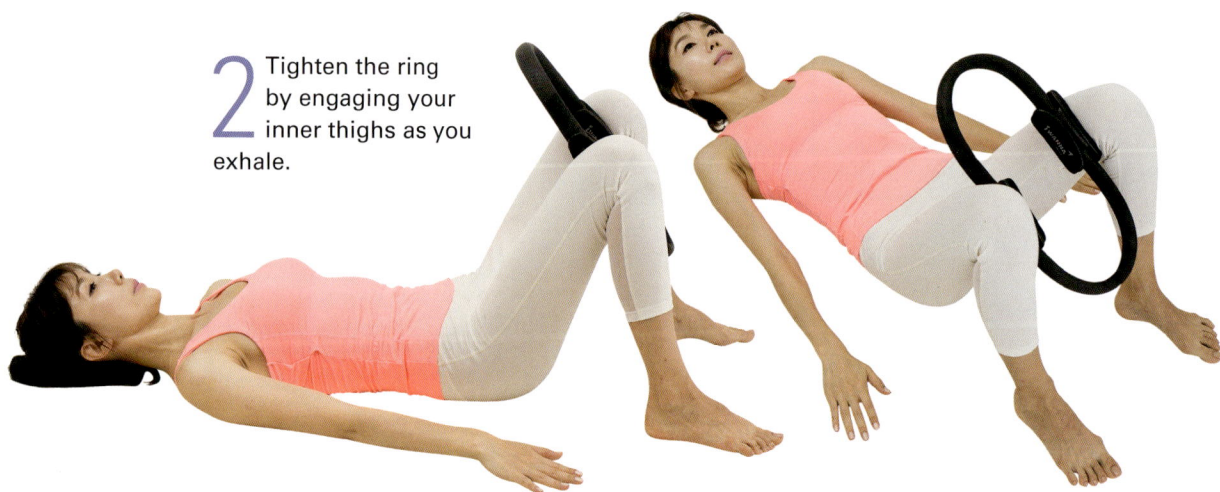

2 Tighten the ring by engaging your inner thighs as you exhale.

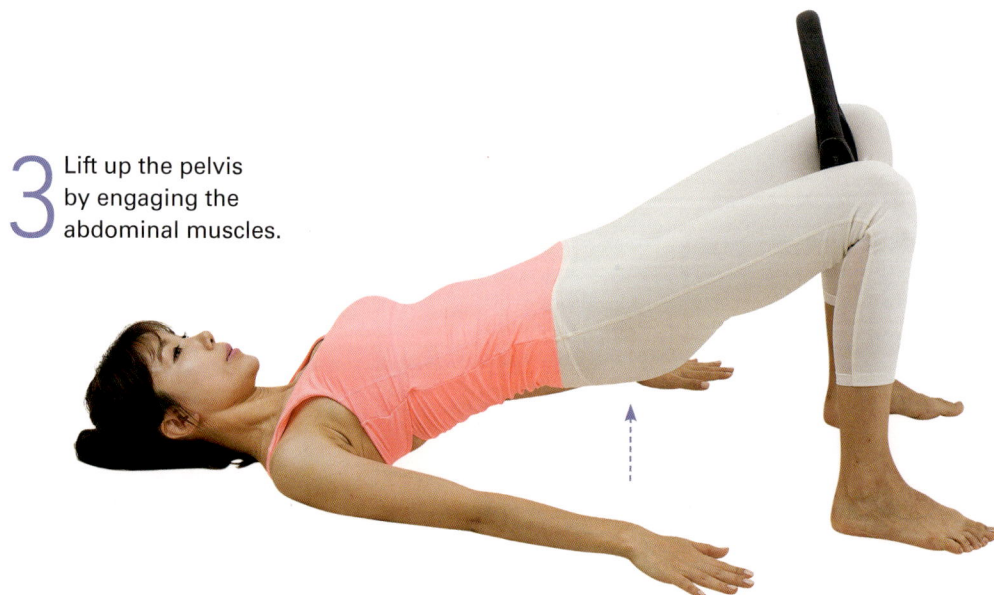

3 Lift up the pelvis by engaging the abdominal muscles.

| The Hundred | This exercise strengthens the abdominal muscles and thighs, while improving core stability and circulation. |

1 Place the ring between your knees and lift up your torso, engaging your abdomen.

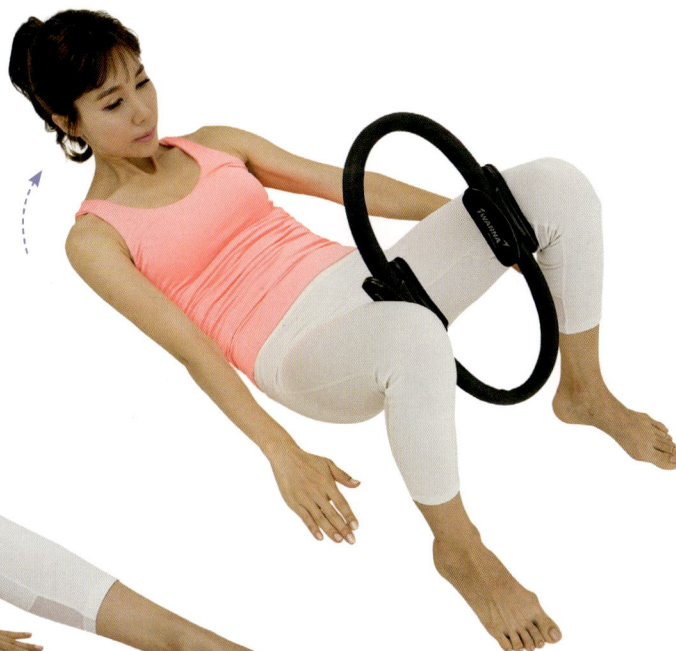

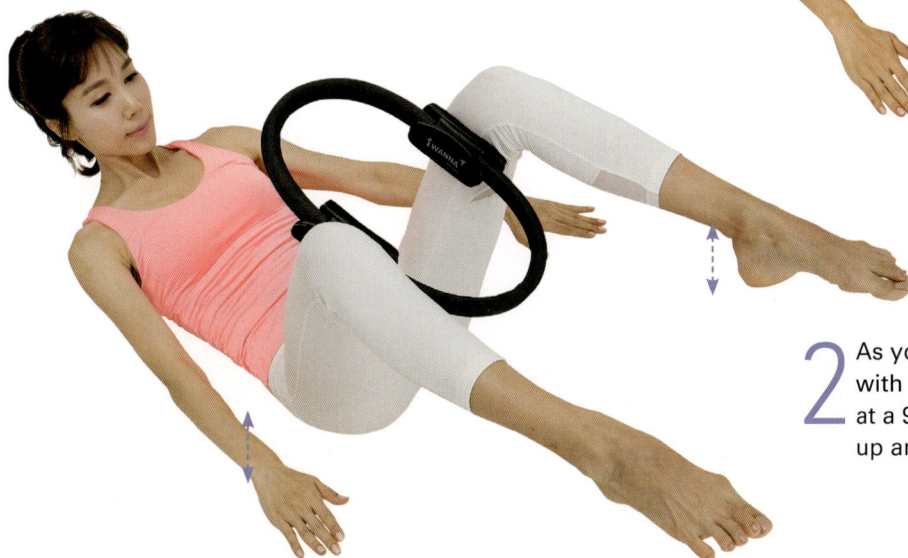

2 As you become more comfortable with the movement, bend your knees at a 90° angle and pump your arms up and down as you breathe.

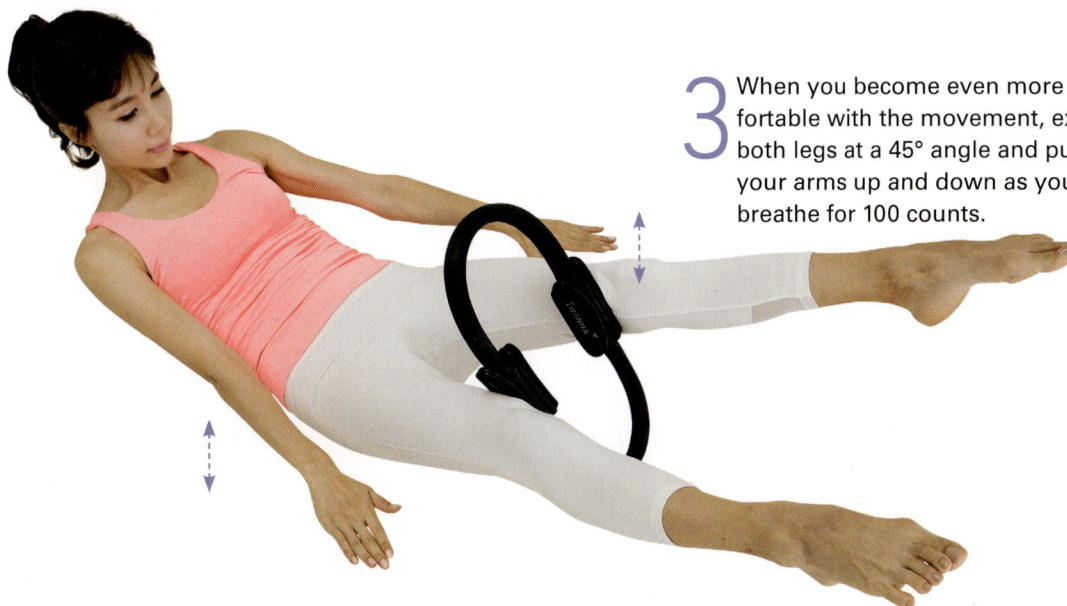

3 When you become even more comfortable with the movement, extend both legs at a 45° angle and pump your arms up and down as you breathe for 100 counts.

This exercise strengthens the core, tones the abdomen, and increases stability.

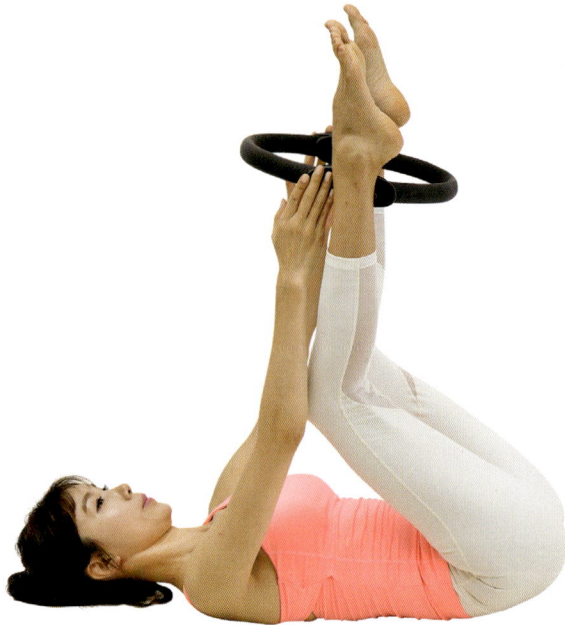

1 Lie on your back with both knees bent at a 90° angle. Place the ring between your ankles.

2 Engage your thighs to keep the ring fixed.

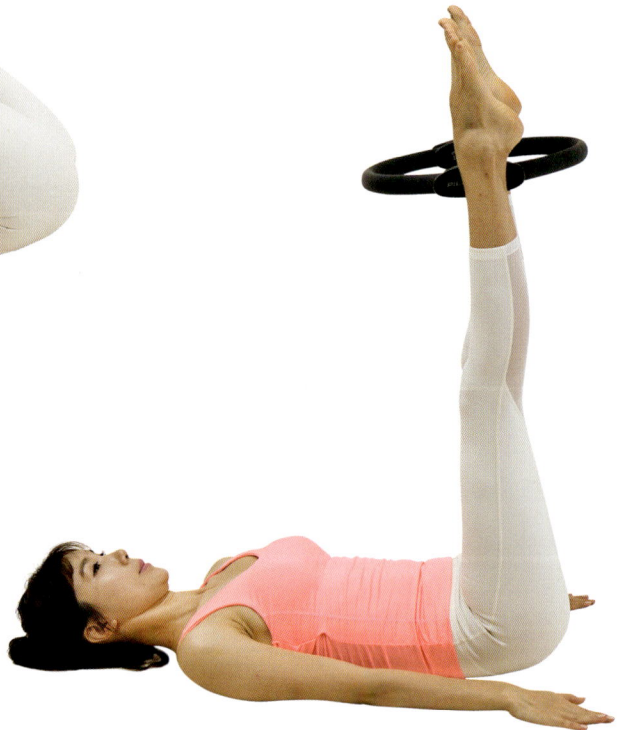

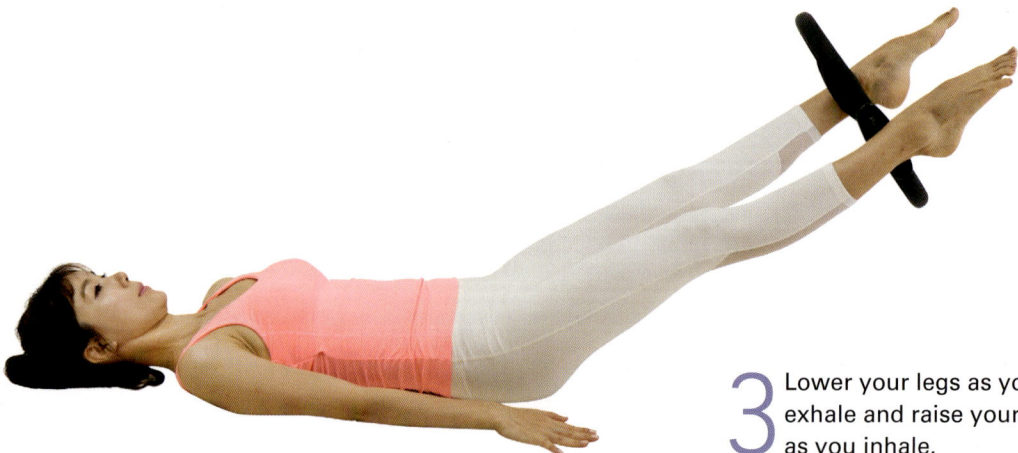

3 Lower your legs as you exhale and raise your legs as you inhale.

| The Teaser | This exercise tones the abdominal area and improves balance. |

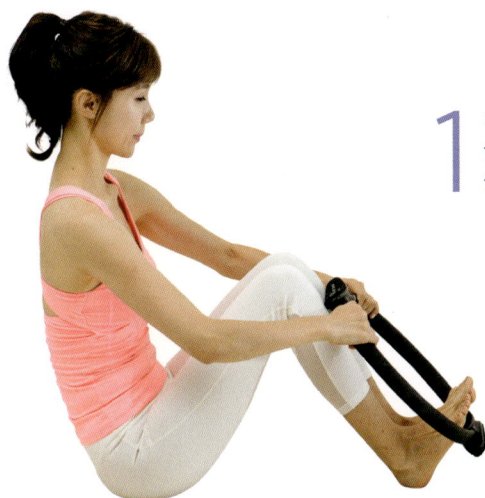

1 Start in a sitting position, then place your feet inside the ring.

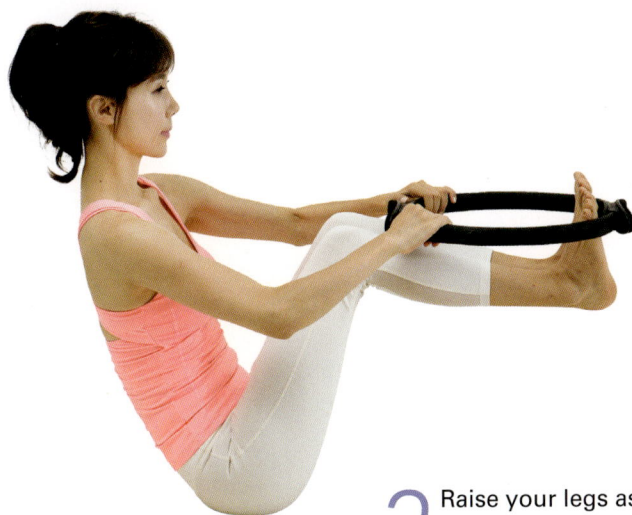

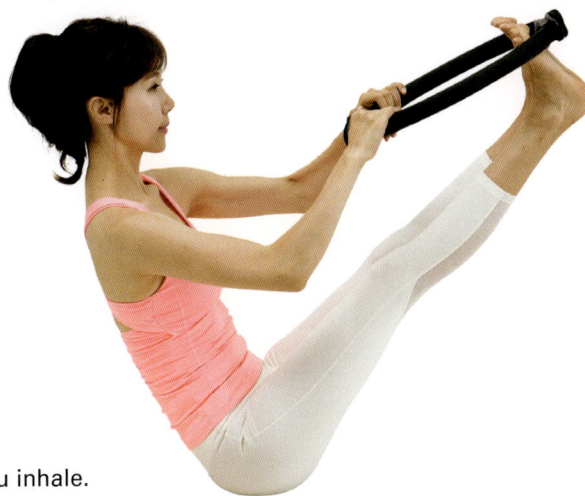

2 Raise your legs as you inhale. Balance while maintaining a V-shape between your torso and legs.

First printed in 2018 in South Korea as Sophia's 필라테스 홈트 by LESSCOM Publishing Company

Published in 2025 in the US by

velopress®

an imprint of The Stable Book Group
32 Court Street, Suite 2109
Brooklyn, NY 11201
www.velopress.com

Library of Congress Control Number: 2025933938
ISBN: 978-1-64604-844-1
eISBN: 978-1-64604-845-8

Photography | Haesung Choi, Bay Studio
Clothes Sponsored by | TrueFoxy (www.truefoxy.com)
Makeup & Hair | Robcosti A.Min

US Editors | Jan Hughes, Renee Rutledge
Design | Haemin Yang
Editor in Chief | Jeanhee Lee
Cover Artwork | background pattern © JTrisno Wardana/shutterstock.com

Printed in China
10 9 8 7 6 5 4 3 2 1

Please Note: This book has been written and published strictly for informational purposes, and in no way
should be used as a substitute for consultation with health care professionals. You should not consider
educational material herein to be the practice of medicine or to replace consultation with a physician or
other medical practitioner. The author and publisher are providing you with information in this work so
that you can have the knowledge and can choose, at your own risk, to act on that knowledge. The author
and publisher also urge all readers to be aware of their health status and to consult health care professionals before beginning any health program.